Accession no.
36172478

McArdle Library APH

B12045

KU-411-436

tma
20/11/13
QV
.4
BAR

Further Essentials of
Pharmacology for Nurses

This book is due for re'

Further Essentials of Pharmacology for Nurses

Paul Barber, Joy Parkes and Diane Blundell

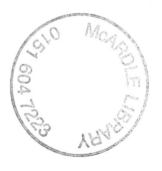

McArdle Library
0151 604 7223

McGraw Hill

Open University Press

Open University Press
McGraw-Hill Education
McGraw-Hill House
Shoppenhangers Road
Maidenhead
Berkshire
England
SL6 2QL

email: enquiries@openup.co.uk
world wide web: www.openup.co.uk

and Two Penn Plaza, New York, NY 10121-2289, USA

First published 2012

Copyright © Paul Barber, Joy Parkes and Diane Blundell, 2012

All rights reserved. Except for the quotation of short passages for the purposes of criticism and review, no part of this publication may be reproduced, stored in a retrieval system, or transmitted, in any form or by any means, electronic, mechanical, photocopying, recording or otherwise, without the prior written permission of the publisher or a licence from the Copyright Licensing Agency Limited. Details of such licences (for reprographic reproduction) may be obtained from the Copyright Licensing Agency Ltd of Saffron House, 6–10 Kirby Street, London, EC1N 8TS.

A catalogue record of this book is available from the British Library

ISBN-13: 9780335243976 (pb)
ISBN-10: 0335243975 (pb)
e-ISBN: 9780335243983

Library of Congress Cataloging-in-Publication Data
CIP data has been applied for

Typeset by Aptara Inc., India
Printed in the UK by Bell and Bain Ltd, Glasgow.

Fictitious names of companies, products, people, characters and/or data that may be used herein (in case studies or in examples) are not intended to represent any real individual, company, product or event.

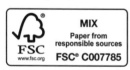

The McGraw·Hill Companies

Praise for this book

"The book provides an easy to follow introductory text for student nurses exploring the world of clinical pharmacology. Each chapter describes the contents and learning outcomes clearly allowing the student to easily navigate to areas they wish to explore. It uses uncomplicated language and case studies and questions that provide students with concrete examples, relating to real life situations, upon which they can develop their pharmacological knowledge and understanding. Clinical tips are clear and illustrate the key points that should be considered by the nurse in the real care giving environment, including acknowledgement of the increasing usage of complementary medicine."

David Armstrong, Senior Lecturer, Northumbria University, UK

"The first book Essentials of Pharmacology for Nurses was an excellent first venture into pharmacology. This new book goes further to explain in more depth specific common disease processes including anatomy and physiology as well as the medications/drugs which may be used. It covers comprehensively the action of drugs, side-effects and other issues that as a nurse you might want to give consideration to. This book would be essential reading for pre-registration nursing students who want to build on their existing knowledge. Other useful aspects are the quizzes, drug calculations and patient scenarios."

Margaret Dilger, Lecturer, University of Salford, UK

Contents

List of abbreviations

ACE	angiotensin-converting enzyme		IV	intravenous
ASA	American Society of Anaesthesiologists		LDL	low-density lipoprotein
			HDL	high-density lipoprotein
ATP	adenosine triphosphate		HMG-CoA	hydroxy-methylglutaryl-coenzyme A
AV	atrioventricular		MAC	minimum alveolar concentration
BBB	blood-brain barrier		MAOI	monoamine oxidase inhibitor
BCG	Bacillus Calmette-Guérin		MHRA	Medicines and Healthcare products Regulatory Agency
BMI	body mass index			
BNF	British National Formulary		MMR	measles, mumps and rubella
BPH	benign prostatic hyperplasia		MRSA	Methicillin-resistant *Staphylococcus aureus*
CAM	complementary and alternative medicine			
			NG	nasogastric
CCK	cholecystokinin		NHS	National Health Service
CHD	coronary heart disease		NICE	National Institute for Health and Clinical Excellence
CSF	cerebral spinal fluid			
CTZ	chemotactic trigger zone		NMB	neuromuscular blocking
CVD	cardiovascular disease		NMDA	N-methyl D-aspartate
DH	Department of Health		NRT	nicotine replacement therapy
DHFR	dihydrofolate reductase		NSAID	non-steroidal anti-inflammatory drug
DHT	dihydrotestosterone		PAF	platelet-activating factor
DNA	deoxyribonucleic acid		PE	pulmonary embolus
EBV	Epstein-Barr virus		PEG	percutaneous endoscopic gastrostomy
ECG	electrocardiogram			
GABA	gamma-aminobutyric acid		PGD	patient group direction
GALT	gut-associated lymphoid tissue		PLN	product licence number
GBE	ginkgo biloba extract		PPI	proton pump inhibitor
GI	gastrointestinal		PSD	patient-specific direction
GLA	gamma-linolenic acid		PT	prothrombin time
GORD	gastro-oesophageal reflux disease		PVC	polyvinylchloride
GTN	glyceryl trinitrate		RCN	Royal College of Nursing
HP	*helicobacter pylori*		RCoA	Royal College of Anaesthetists
HPC	Health Professions Council		RNA	ribonucleic acid
HPV	human papilloma virus		SA	sinoatrial
HRT	hormone replacement therapy		SC	subcutaneous
IBS	irritable bowel syndrome		SSRI	selective serotonin reuptake inhibitor
IH	inhaled		TB	tuberculosis
IM	intramuscular		THR	traditional herbal registration
INR	International Normalized Ratio		TIVA	total IV anaesthesia

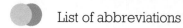

TPN	total parenteral nutrition	VF	ventricular fibrillation
TSM	transparent semi-permeable membrane	VLDL	very low density lipoprotein
		VT	ventricular tachycardia

Introduction

Firstly, thank you if you purchased a copy of the first book, *Essentials of Pharmacology for Nurses* by Barber and Robertson (Open University Press 2009, with a new edition published in 2012). This second book is written in an attempt to build on that volume by focusing on more specific and specialized medicines. You will have now begun to appreciate the foundations of the subject in relation to nursing. It is now time to take the journey further. This book has some of the same features as the first, in that it will bring to life and engage you in the subjects of pharmacology and calculation of drug dosage. Some chapters have been enhanced by the inclusion of relevant aspects of physiology.

It is worth mentioning that because of their specific nature some drugs will not be administered by a nurse (e.g. general anaesthetic agents and complementary medicines). However, it is important for the student to have an understanding of the impact of these drugs from a nursing perspective.

As in the last book, we have included drug calculations where applicable. However, the book does not contain detailed formulae – rather it gives you a basic structure on which to build. We wanted the calculations to reflect each of the chapters' content (where applicable) and to give you a sense of what might be expected in practice. In the first two chapters we have given you the method of working for each answer to build your confidence: after that we felt you should be able to do the maths yourself. Calculations are well covered in other texts, some of which you will find in the recommended further reading section at the end of each chapter. These sections deliberately repeat the key texts in this field for your ease of reference, and in addition include works specific to the chapter's topic.

A further feature we retain in this book is the inclusion of case studies and, unlike most other books, we have included examples of some of the points that you should have been considering in analysing these scenarios.

Where possible we have also tried to focus the pharmacology on nursing practice. You will notice that each chapter contains boxes entitled 'Clinical tip'. These should assist you in reflecting on your everyday practice.

Finally, we have included multiple choice questions for each of the chapters. All the questions are based on information included in the chapter and we hope you enjoy getting them all right!

Well dear student, it is now time to embark on the next step of what we hope will be a fascinating journey. Don't forget that the key to your learning is the level of your motivation. Enjoy!

1

Cardiovascular drugs

Chapter contents

Learning objectives

After studying this chapter you should be able to:

- Briefly explain the epidemiology and aetiology of cardiovascular disease in the UK.
- Describe what is meant by atherosclerosis.
- Demonstrate an understanding of the role of cholesterol in the body.
- List the principal drug categories used in lowering cholesterol levels.
- Describe what is meant by the term 'angina'.
- Outline how nitrate drugs affect the body.
- Explain electrical conduction through the heart.
- Review the physiology of cardiac muscle contraction.
- Describe the terms 'paroxysmal', 'supraventricular', 'tachycardia' and 'atrial fibrillation'.

- Compare and contrast the modes of action between different drug classifications used in the treatment of arrhythmias.
- Outline the drugs used in cardiopulmonary resuscitation.
- Demonstrate what you understand about the condition Wolff-Parkinson-White syndrome.
- Use basic maths to calculate simple drug dosages.

Introduction

Cardiovascular disease (CVD) causes more deaths in the UK each year than any other single disease or condition. According to the British Heart Foundation (2011) CVD costs the National Health Service (NHS) nearly £15 billion annually. Coronary heart disease (CHD) is preventable and yet was the cause of 18 per cent of male and 12 per cent of female deaths in 2009. Between 110,000 and 300,000 people have a heart attack each year.

The problem of CHD does not stop with the death rate but includes the symptoms of angina. Angina is chest pain or discomfort that occurs when an area of the heart muscle does not receive enough oxygen-rich blood. It may feel like pressure or squeezing in the chest and/or like indigestion. The pain may also occur in the shoulders, arms, neck, jaw or back. Angina affects about 1 in 50 people, and in the UK there are between 1.2 and 2 million sufferers (British Heart Foundation 2011). It affects men more than women, and your chances of suffering from angina increase as you get older. The pain resulting from angina and the consequent restriction on lifestyle causes a great reduction in quality of life.

Senior (2010) suggests that the stereotypical view that we tend to have of heart disease is that it affects middle-aged men. Women are thought to be much less likely to have a heart attack and it is therefore a sobering fact that three times as many women die of heart disease than of breast cancer each year in the UK. Although the female hormones do provide some protection against heart disease before the menopause, the growing impact of risk factors such as an unhealthy diet, smoking and taking too little exercise means that a higher proportion of younger women are now succumbing to heart disease. Following the menopause, the lack of oestrogen – and therefore the loss of its protective benefits – increases a woman's risk of CVD to the same level as a man's.

Senior goes on to highlight that although younger people are now developing chronic heart disease earlier in life, the UK figures for congenital heart disease show that fewer than 5000 babies born in any one year suffer a problem with their heart, such as a hole in the heart. Surgical treatments for congenital heart problems are very advanced in the UK and survival rates are high.

The underlying cause of heart disease in the UK is lifestyle. We just do not live healthy lives. Many people in the UK are overweight – around 43 per cent of adult men and 32 per cent of adult women. Worse still, 30 per cent of children are overweight and experts predict that heart disease in the future will continue to rise. Younger people now have the same sorts of problems with their cardiovascular system as middle-aged people did a few years ago.

The number of people who have other risk factors for heart disease is also high: 6 out of 10 people over 18 in the UK have high cholesterol, approximately 30 per cent of all adults have high blood pressure and far less than half of all adults take enough exercise. Smoking continues to be a habit which kills 25,000 people every year because of the impact it has on the cardiovascular system. Most of these deaths could have been prevented.

Most nurses will care for a person suffering from heart disease of some form, and therefore it is of great importance that we understand the medicines they take in order to afford them the best quality care.

Atherosclerosis

Atheroma is the root cause of cardiovascular diseases such as angina and heart attack. However, before we delve into the pathophysiology of this type of disease we need to revisit the anatomy and physiology of the blood vessels.

The walls of all blood vessels, apart from capillaries, have the same basic layers or 'tunics'. The outermost layer is called the *tunica adventitia* and is composed of fibrous connective tissue. The middle layer is known as the *tunica media* and is made up predominantly of smooth muscle. Finally the inner layer is referred to as the *tunica intima* and comprises flattened epithelial cells. This inner layer of the vessel is also referred to as the *endothelium*. The endothelium works to keep the inside of arteries toned and smooth, which keeps blood flowing.

Atherosclerosis is a degenerative disease that results in narrowing of the arteries. It is caused by fatty deposits, most notably cholesterol, on the interior walls of the coronary arteries. When the walls become narrowed or occluded, the blood flow through the artery is reduced (see Figure 1.1). When this occurs in the coronary arteries the blood flow to the heart muscle is reduced. If the artery remains open to some degree, the reduced blood flow is noticed during periods of rapid heartbeat. The resulting pain is called angina. When the artery is completely closed or occluded, a section of the heart muscle can no longer get oxygenated blood, and begins to die. This is called a heart attack or *myocardial infarction*. Only quickly restoring the blood flow can reduce the amount of heart muscle that will die.

Cholesterol

Cholesterol is a waxy, fat-like (lipid) substance that is found in all cells of the body. In addition to being a structural component of cell membranes, cholesterol also plays an important role in making hormones, vitamin D and bile acids that aid in the digestion of foods. Cholesterol itself is not harmful, but too much cholesterol in the blood, or high blood cholesterol, can be dangerous. Blood is watery, and cholesterol is fatty. Just like oil and water, the two do not mix. To travel in the bloodstream, cholesterol is carried in small packages called *lipoproteins*. There are two kinds of lipoprotein that carry cholesterol throughout the body: low-density lipoprotein (LDL) and high-density lipoprotein (HDL).

- LDL is the main cholesterol transporter and carries cholesterol from your liver to the cells that need it. If there is too much cholesterol for the cells to use, this can cause a harmful build-up in your blood. Too much LDL cholesterol in the blood can cause cholesterol to build up in the artery walls, leading to disease of the arteries. For this reason, LDL cholesterol is known as 'bad cholesterol', and lower levels are preferable.
- HDL carries cholesterol *away* from the cells and back to the liver, where it is either broken down or passed from the body as a waste product. For this reason, it is referred to as 'good cholesterol', and higher levels are preferable.

The amount of cholesterol in the blood (including both LDL and HDL) can be measured with a blood test.

Normal cholesterol level

Blood cholesterol is measured in units called millimoles per litre of blood, often shortened to mmol/L. The Department of Health (DH) recommends that cholesterol levels should be less than 5mmol/L. In the UK, two out of three adults have a total cholesterol level of 5mmol/L or above. On

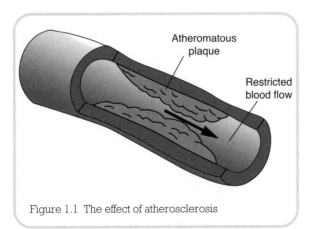

Figure 1.1 The effect of atherosclerosis

Atheromatous plaque

Restricted blood flow

average, men in England have a cholesterol level of 5.5mmol/L and women have a level of 5.6mmol/L. The UK population has one of the highest average cholesterol concentrations in the world.

Diets that are high in saturated fats and cholesterol raise the levels of LDL cholesterol in the blood. Fats are classified as 'saturated' or 'unsaturated' according to their chemical structure. Saturated fats are derived primarily from meat and dairy products and can raise blood cholesterol levels. Some vegetable oils made from coconut, palm and cocoa are also high in saturated fats.

Lowering LDL cholesterol is currently the primary focus in preventing atherosclerosis and heart attacks. Lowering LDL involves losing excess weight, exercising regularly and following a diet that is low in saturated fat and cholesterol. Medications are prescribed when lifestyle changes cannot reduce the LDL cholesterol to desired levels. The most effective and widely used medications to lower LDL cholesterol are called statins. Most of the large controlled trials that demonstrated the benefits of lowering LDL cholesterol in the prevention of myocardial infarction and cerebrovascular accident used one of the statins.

Lipid regulating drugs

Lowering the amount of LDLs and raising the levels of HDLs slows the progression of atherosclerosis and may even cause a reduction in its formation. However, before medication is considered in people who are deemed to be at high risk of cardiovascular disease, changes in lifestyle should be advised. These lifestyle changes include changes to the diet, particularly in terms of fat and salt content. An increase in exercise is an important step and many GPs work with local councils in offering exercise regimes for free, or at a reduced fee, to encourage participation. Smoking and alcohol consumption are further areas of lifestyle that require modification in order for the individual to lower their chances of developing cardiovascular disease.

Statins

Statins lower the level of cholesterol in the blood by reducing the production of cholesterol by the liver. Statins block the enzyme in the liver that is responsible for making cholesterol. This enzyme is called hydroxy-methylglutaryl-coenzyme A reductase (HMG-CoA reductase). Scientifically, statins are referred to as 'HMG-CoA reductase inhibitors' and you should be aware that some pharmacology texts index this class of drug under this name rather than an index heading of 'statins'.

This class of drug reduces the risk of cardiovascular disease, irrespective of the cholesterol content of the blood. This makes statins the drug of first choice for primary and secondary prevention of cardiovascular disease. By 'primary prevention' we mean they help prevent significant build-up of atheroma so that cardiovascular disease can be avoided. Secondary prevention relates to a reduction in cardiovascular disease once the person has already been diagnosed or had an 'event', such as angina or myocardial infarction.

Most individuals are placed on statins because of high levels of cholesterol. Though reduction of cholesterol is important, heart disease is complex. Thirty-five per cent of individuals who develop heart attacks do not have high blood cholesterol levels, yet most of them have atherosclerosis. This means that high levels of cholesterol are not always necessary for atherosclerotic deposits or plaques to form.

Because it is not clear which effect of statins is responsible for their benefits, the goal of treatment with this drug should not only be the reduction of cholesterol to normal levels, but also the prevention of the complications of atherosclerosis (angina, heart attacks, stroke, intermittent claudication and death). This is important because it allows for individuals who have, or are at risk of, atherosclerosis but who do not have high levels of cholesterol, to be considered for treatment with statins.

Statins are usually well absorbed, given orally and prescribed last thing before going to bed. One of the most obvious differences between different statins is the ability to reduce cholesterol. Currently, atorvastatin (Lipitor) and rosuvastatin (Crestor) are the most potent, and fluvastatin (Lescol) is the least potent.

The statins also differ in how strongly they interact with other drugs. Specifically, pravastatin (Pravachol) and rosuvastatin (Crestor) levels in the body are less likely to be elevated by other drugs that may be taken at the same time as statins. This is so because the enzymes in the liver that eliminate pravastatin and rosuvastatin are not blocked by many of the drugs that block the enzymes that eliminate other statins. This is referred to in technical terms as 'enzyme inhibition' and is discussed in Chapter 2 of *Essentials of Pharmacology for Nurses* (Barber and Robertson 2012). This in turn prevents the levels of pravastatin and rosuvastatin from rising and leading to increased toxicity which results in myopathy (inflammation of the muscles).

The most serious (but fortunately rare) side-effects of statins are liver failure and rhabdomyolysis. Rhabdomyolysis is a serious side-effect in which there is damage to the muscles and involves the breakdown of muscle fibres, resulting in the release of myoglobins into the bloodstream, some of which are harmful to the kidneys and frequently result in damage to those organs. Rhabdomyolysis often begins as muscle pain and can progress to loss of muscle cells, kidney failure and death. It occurs more often when statins are used in combination with other drugs that themselves cause rhabdomyolysis such as selective serotonin reuptake inhibitors (SSRIs), or with drugs that prevent the elimination of statins and raise the levels of statins in the blood.

> **Clinical tip**
>
> Since rhabdomyolysis may be fatal, unexplained joint or muscle pain that occurs while taking statins should be taken seriously by the nurse, documented and passed on to the doctor for evaluation. Statins must not be used during pregnancy because of the risk of serious adverse effects to the developing foetus.

Since the primary effects of statins are on the liver it is clear that any problems with the liver would cause concern when prescribing such medicines. Indeed, statins should be used with caution in those with liver disease or with a high alcohol intake. The National Institute for Health and Clinical Excellence (NICE) guideline 67 suggests that liver enzymes should be measured before treatment and that measurement should be repeated within 3 months and at the end of 12 months after starting treatment.

Fibrates

Fibrates are a class of medication that lowers blood triglyceride levels by reducing the production in the liver of very low density lipoproteins (VLDLs) (the triglyceride-carrying particles that circulate in the blood) and by speeding up the removal of triglycerides from the blood. Raised levels of triglycerides are often part of what is known as 'metabolic syndrome', a condition that increases the risk of cardiovascular disease. A person with metabolic syndrome will have excess weight around the waist and at least two of the following:

- high blood pressure;
- raised levels of triglycerides;
- low levels of HDL cholesterol;
- abnormal fasting blood glucose.

However, researchers are increasingly recognizing that raised triglycerides can by themselves increase the risk of cardiovascular disease, even if cholesterol levels are normal.

Fibrates are also modestly effective in increasing blood HDL cholesterol levels; however, they are not effective in lowering LDL cholesterol. Examples of fibrates available in the UK include gemfibrozil (Lopid) and fenofibrate (Lipantil).

Even though fibrates are not effective in lowering LDL cholesterol, when a high-risk patient also has high blood triglyceride or low HDL cholesterol levels doctors may consider combining a fibrate, such as fenofibrate (Lipantil) with a statin. Such a combination will not only lower LDL cholesterol but will also lower blood triglycerides and increase HDL cholesterol levels.

Bile-acid binding resins

Bile-acid binding resins, and similar agents including powders such as cholestyramine (Questran and Questran Light) and tablet preparations like colesevelam hydrochloride (Cholestagel) are able to lower LDL. As their name suggests, they work by binding to bile in the digestive tract. As part of normal digestion, the liver turns cholesterol into bile acids and these move into the intestines, where most of them are reabsorbed and returned to the liver. Bile-acid drugs bind to the bile acids as they move through the intestine so that the acids exit the body with the faeces, rather than re-entering the bloodstream. In response, the liver converts more cholesterol into bile acids and these, too, are cleared from the body in the faeces. The result is that LDL cholesterol is effectively removed from the liver and the blood.

When used with dietary control, bile-acid resins can reduce LDL levels by 15–20 per cent. When they are combined with nicotinic acid, LDL levels can drop by as much as 40–60 per cent. Colesevelam, a newer resin, appears to produce minimal gastrointestinal (GI) side-effects.

Clinical tip

Patients often experience constipation, heartburn, gas and other GI problems while taking a drug in this class and so it is important that you explain these potential side-effects to the patient prior to their commencing therapy. These symptoms can become so bothersome that the person may seek to change, or cease to take, their medication.

Over time, deficiencies of vitamins A, D, E, K and B9 (folic acid) may occur, and vitamin supplements may be necessary. If long-term use of bile-acid binding resins leads to depletion of vitamin K in the body, problems of bleeding may occur.

Rarely, toxic effects on the liver have been reported and therefore patients with liver disorders should always be monitored. Bile-acid binding resins may interfere with other medications, including digoxin, warfarin, beta-blocker drugs for high blood pressure (such as atenolol, metoprolol and propranolol), diuretics and sulfonylureas (such as glimepiride), used to treat diabetes. In order to prevent these adverse interactions, such medications should be taken one hour before, or four to six hours after, taking the bile-acid binding resin.

Angina

Angina (*angina pectoris*, Latin for 'squeezing of the chest') is discomfort that occurs when there is a decreased blood oxygen supply to an area of the heart muscle. In most cases, the lack of blood supply is due to a narrowing of the coronary arteries as a result of atherosclerosis.

Angina usually occurs during exertion, severe emotional stress or after a heavy meal. During these periods the heart muscle demands more blood oxygen than the narrowed coronary arteries can deliver. Angina typically lasts from 1 to 15 minutes and is classified as either stable or unstable.

Stable angina is the most common type, and what most people mean when they refer to 'angina'. People with stable angina suffer angina symptoms on a regular basis and the symptoms are somewhat predictable (e.g. walking up a flight of steps causes chest pain). For most patients, symptoms occur during exertion and commonly last less than five minutes. They are relieved by rest or medication such as glyceryl trinitrate under the tongue (sublingual).

Unstable angina is now referred to as 'acute coronary syndrome' and is less common and more serious. The symptoms are more severe and less predictable and the pains are more frequent, last longer, occur at rest and are not relieved by glyceryl trinitrate. Unstable angina is not the same as a heart attack, but warrants an immediate visit to a GP or hospital emergency department as further cardiac testing is urgently needed. Unstable angina often precedes myocardial infarction.

Glyceryl trinitrate

The first drug to be considered in the relief of angina is glyceryl trinitrate, more commonly known as GTN, which belongs to a group of drugs called nitrates that contain the chemical nitric oxide. This chemical is made naturally by the body and has the effect of making the veins and arteries relax and widen (dilate). As a result more oxygen can be carried in the blood and the heart does not have to work so hard to keep up with both the demands of the tissues and the resistance caused by the atheroma in the vessels.

Widening the veins also decreases the volume of blood that returns to the heart with each heartbeat (preload). This makes it easier for the heart to pump that blood out again. As a result of both of these actions, the heart does not need as much energy to pump the blood around the body and therefore needs less oxygen. GTN also widens the arteries within the heart itself, which increases the blood and oxygen supply to the heart muscle.

This drug can be prescribed in a variety of forms, including tablets and an oral spray. The tablets are designed to be slow release and dissolve under the tongue. They usually come in a dose of 300mcg per tablet. The spray is also applied under the tongue, as this area is highly vascular, meaning that there is a plentiful supply of blood vessels that can absorb the medication. The spray gives a dose of 400mcg per dose. This drug is ingested sublingually because if it were swallowed it would be absorbed by blood vessels that go straight to the liver. This drug is broken down very rapidly by the liver (the 'first pass' effect) and as a result, following the first pass through the liver there would not be enough active drug remaining to be of any use in preventing the episode of angina.

The drug effect starts rapidly, usually within one minute of administration and lasts between 15 and 30 minutes. Patients often have a choice of which preparation they prefer and the drug can be taken on an 'as required' basis, which benefits the patient if they anticipate doing any exercise or activity that will put additional pressure and workload on the heart.

As GTN is absorbed well by the skin it is also available in transdermal patches – medicated adhesive pads that are placed on the skin to deliver a time-release dose of medication into the bloodstream. Therapeutic levels of the drug are achieved in approximately 1 hour and last for a period of 24 hours.

Clinical tip

One of the problems with using GTN tablets is that once a bottle has been opened the drug effects start to deteriorate (short shelf life). Therefore it is important that the patient does not hoard the drug over a period of time, as it will become ineffective. Spray preparations overcome this problem and are therefore gaining in popularity.

Clinical tip

Using transdermal patches safely and effectively

DO NOT

- Shave the area.
- Apply a new patch without first removing the previously applied patch.
- Get any medication on your hands or touch the adhesive surface of the patch.
- Apply a patch to damaged or irritated skin or to an area with skin folds or scars.
- Apply a patch below your patient's elbows or knees.

DO

- Take your patient's vital signs and check other assessment parameters, as indicated, such as pain scoring.
- Explain to your patient that the patch contains a medication. Tell them about the drug, its purpose and possible adverse effects.
- Check any expiry date to ensure the patch is within date.
- Wash your hands and put on gloves.
- Select a clean, dry area of skin such as the upper chest. Clip body hair, if necessary.
- Clean the selected area according to the manufacturer's directions.
- Remove the patch from its protective covering. Without touching the adhesive, remove the clear plastic backing.
- Use your palm to apply the patch and press firmly for about 10 seconds. Check that the patch adheres well, especially around the edges. Write the date, the time and the site used in the patient's records.
- Remove the patch for a few hours in every 24 to avoid the patient building up a tolerance to glyceryl trinitrate.
- Remove the used patch and dispose of it safely – it contains residual medication that could harm others, particularly children or pets.
- Reapply the transdermal patch at the correct time to ensure the appropriate medication effect. To avoid irritating the patient's skin, rotate application sites, using the corresponding site on the opposite side of the patient's body. Try not to use the same site more than once a week, if possible.

The intravenous (IV) form of GTN is more effective than the sublingual form in controlling arrhythmias arising during acute ischaemic episodes because of prompt delivery of the drug to the coronary circulation where vasodilation occurs. In addition, the ability to control the quantity and rate of drug delivery with an IV infusion offers distinct advantages in cases of coronary spasm occurring during situations such as coronary arteriography where it can be administered with careful electrocardiographic and haemodynamic monitoring.

Clinical tip

It is important to remember that when giving this drug as an infusion you use a syringe pump.

GTN can interact with certain polyvinylchloride (PVC) containers and giving sets. It is not compatible with PVC and severe losses of GTN (up to 50 per cent) may occur if PVC is used, resulting in a reduction of delivered dose and efficacy. Contact of the solution with PVC bags should therefore be avoided.

Clinical tip

GTN is best administered from a glass container and given via a polyethylene giving set.

Isosorbide mononitrate and dinitrate

These are both nitrate drugs and their mode of action is the same as that of GTN, but they have a longer period of action. They are taken in order to prevent, or at least reduce, the occurrence of angina. These drugs will not be effective in a person who is having an angina attack. Side-effects are similar to those of GTN. Isosorbide mononitrate can cause severe headaches, especially when the

Box 1.1 GTN side-effects and interventions

Common side-effects (affect less than 1 in 10 people who take this medicine)	Possible interventions
Light-headedness or dizziness, especially when getting up from a sitting or lying position	Getting up slowly should help. If the patient begins to feel dizzy, suggest they lie down so that they do not faint, then ask them to sit for a few moments before standing
Headache	Patients should inform their doctor who may recommend a suitable painkiller
Dizziness	Make sure the patient understands the importance of their reactions being normal before driving, operating machinery or doing other jobs which could be dangerous
Fast or fluttering heartbeat, feeling sick and flushing	The patient should make an appointment with their doctor

patient first starts taking the drug. However, these may gradually become less severe over time.

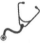

Clinical tip

In the case of headache, the patient should be informed not to stop taking isosorbide mononitrate and to ask a doctor before using any headache pain medication.

Isosorbide dinitrate should not be prescribed if the patient is taking sildenafil (Viagra) as serious, life-threatening side-effects can occur. This is because Viagra can potentiate the vasodilatory effect of isosorbide mononitrate with the potential result of serious syncope (transient loss of consciousness due to a sudden fall in blood pressure) or myocardial infarction.

This medication should not be used if the patient is allergic to isosorbide dinitrate, isosorbide mononitrate (Imdur, ISMO, Monoket) or nitroglycerin, or if there are early signs of a myocardial infarction such as chest pain or 'heavy feeling', pain spreading to the arm or shoulder, nausea, sweating or a general ill feeling.

Tolerance is an issue with nitrate-based drugs and means that following repeated ingestion of a drug the effect produced by the original dose no longer occurs. As a result the dose has to be continually increased to obtain the desired response. It is well documented that people build up a tolerance to this group of drugs and it is therefore important that patients receive a 'nitrate-free period' where the levels of nitrate in the bloodstream are allowed to fall. Such a period should occur every 24 hours.

Finally, you will not find isosorbide dinitrate being used in children as its safety and effectiveness have not been confirmed.

Clinical tip

If a patient has a transdermal patch, advise them to remove it for a six-hour period every day. If a patient is taking three doses of the drug daily it is important to tell them to take the evening tablet at teatime rather than before going to bed.

The next group of drugs is those used when the heart has been damaged and, as a result, the rhythm of the organ has been altered. This group, not surprisingly, is called *anti-arrhythmic* medicines. First, however, it is important to remind ourselves about the processes involved in the contraction of the heart muscle and the electrical conduction through the heart, as a number of anti-arrhythmic medicines act on these.

Electrical conduction through the heart

The heart is a muscle with a special electrical conduction system. The system is made up of two nodes (special conduction cells) and a series of conduction fibres or bundles (pathways).

The normal heart begins with an electrical impulse from the sinoatrial (SA) node, located high in the right atrium (number 1 in Figure 1.2). The SA node is the pacemaker of the normal heart, responsible for setting the rate and rhythm. The impulse spreads through the walls of the atria, causing them to contract. Next, the impulse moves through the atrioventricular (AV) node, a relay

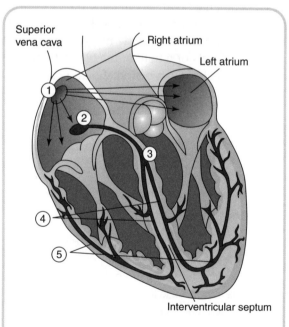

Figure 1.2 Electrical conduction through the heart

station (number 2), into the 'bundle of His' (number 3), continuing into conduction bundles (numbers 4 and 5) which are located in the ventricles themselves. As the impulse travels down the bundles, the ventricles contract. The cycle then repeats itself.

This regular cycle of atrial and ventricular contractions pumps blood effectively out of the heart. Problems may occur anywhere in the conduction system and interfere with effective pumping of blood. The heart may beat too fast (tachycardia), too slow (bradycardia) or irregularly. These abnormal beats are known as arrhythmias. Special studies of the heart's electrical system may be needed to accurately diagnose the type and cause of the arrhythmia. Therapy for arrhythmias is based on their type and the difficulties they cause.

Contraction of cardiac muscle

To look at, cardiac muscle is similar to skeletal (striated) muscle. However, cardiac muscle differs from skeletal muscle in the membranes that separate each muscle. Cardiac muscles are separated by what are known as *intercalated discs*. The discs have a very low electrical resistance which means that the *action potential*, or *wave of contraction*, can spread throughout the cardiac muscle very easily. This means that the heart muscle can act as a functional whole as soon as it is excited. Given that the heart acts as a pump, this is of prime importance.

If you have read Chapter 3 of *Essentials of Pharmacology for Nurses* (Barber and Robertson 2012) on local anaesthetics and analgesics, you will appreciate the importance of understanding the movement of ions across membranes. This appreciation comes into play once again when discussing cardiac contraction. In order for the myocardium to contract, sodium must enter the muscle cell. This is known as Phase 0 of the action potential or *depolarization* (contraction). Phase 1 occurs next, where the movement of sodium ions into the muscle ceases and potassium ions start to move out. The heart muscle is getting ready to fire again (*repolarization*). Phase 2 is very important in terms of muscular contraction of the heart and is known as the *plateau*. In this phase the potassium

In the figure, the following labels appear: Superior vena cava, Right atrium, Left atrium, and Interventricular septum, with numbered points 1, 2, 3, 4, 5.

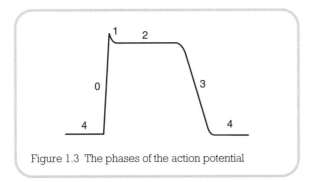

Figure 1.3 The phases of the action potential

ions continue to move out of the muscle cell but this is counterbalanced by a slow inward movement of calcium ions. This phase helps with heart contraction by slowing the rate of repolarization. Phase 3 continues the further movement of potassium ions out of the cardiac muscle. Phase 4 is said to have been reached by the swapping of potassium and sodium across the membrane so that it is ready to receive another action potential and the cycle starts all over again (see Figure 1.3).

Drugs used in heart arrhythmias

Anti-arrhythmic drugs can be grouped under three headings:

- drugs that act on supraventricular arrhythmias (originating above the ventricles);
- drugs that act on both supraventricular and ventricular arrhythmias;
- drugs that act on ventricular arrhythmias (originating in the ventricles).

Before we go on to consider these drugs in more detail it is worth noting that all anti-arrhythmic drugs have potentially serious side-effects. They may worsen or indeed cause life-threatening arrhythmias themselves. Close medical and nursing monitoring is therefore essential.

Paroxysmal supraventricular tachycardia

Paroxysmal supraventricular tachycardia is a regular, fast (160 to 220 beats per minute) heart rate that begins and ends suddenly and originates in heart tissue other than that of the ventricles. It is most common among young people, is more unpleasant than dangerous and may occur during vigorous exercise.

The fast heart rate may last from a few minutes to many hours. It is almost always experienced as an uncomfortable palpitation. It is often associated with other symptoms such as weakness, lightheadedness, shortness of breath and chest pain. Usually, the heart is otherwise normal. The doctor confirms the diagnosis by doing an electrocardiogram (ECG).

Episodes of paroxysmal supraventricular tachycardia can often be prevented by one of several manoeuvres that stimulate the vagus nerve and thus decrease the heart rate. The heart rate decreases because the vagus nerve initiates a parasympathetic effect. These manoeuvres are usually conducted or supervised by a doctor, but people who repeatedly experience the arrhythmia often learn to perform them themselves. In practice you may see the doctor rubbing the neck just below the angle of the jaw; this stimulates a sensitive area on the carotid artery called the carotid sinus. This is a dilated area located at the junction where the carotid arteries split (bifurcate) and contains numerous baroreceptors that function in the control of blood pressure by influencing changes in the heart rate. If this is not effective, if the arrhythmia produces severe symptoms, or if the episode lasts more than 20 minutes, doctors can usually stop an episode promptly by giving an IV injection, usually of adenosine.

Adenosine

Adenosine is a compound that occurs naturally in all cells of the body. One of its properties is to slow down the electrical impulses through a specialized area of tissue in the heart – the AV node – in order to attempt to restore a normal heart rate and rhythm (sinus rhythm) when a person is having an episode of paroxysmal supraventricular tachycardia.

The drug is administered by rapid IV bolus injection and is intended for hospital use only, with monitoring and cardiorespiratory resuscitation equipment available for immediate use.

Clinical tip

To be certain the solution reaches the systemic circulation the adenosine should be administered either directly into a vein or into an IV line. If administered via an IV line it should be injected as near as possible to the patient and followed by a rapid saline flush. The drug should only be used when facilities for cardiac monitoring exist.

An adult may receive an initial dose of 3mg given as a rapid IV injection over a two-second period. If the patient's heart rhythm does not respond then a second dose of 6mg should be given. If this is not successful then a third dose of 12mg can be considered. The drug can be used in children but, as you would expect, the dose is smaller: between 0.0375 and 0.25mg/kg.

Atrial fibrillation

Atrial fibrillation is a condition where the heart's two upper chambers (the atria) beat chaotically and irregularly – out of coordination with the two lower chambers (the ventricles). Atrial fibrillation is an irregular and often rapid heart rate that commonly causes poor blood flow to the body and symptoms of heart palpitations, shortness of breath and weakness. It can also cause fatigue and stroke. This condition is often caused by changes in the heart that occur as a result of heart disease. Episodes of atrial fibrillation can come and go, or a patient may have chronic atrial fibrillation. If the latter is the case, because the atria are beating rapidly and irregularly, blood does not flow through them as quickly. This makes the blood more likely to clot. If the clot is pumped out of the heart it can travel to the brain (cerebral embolism), resulting in a stroke. People with atrial fibrillation are five to seven times more likely to have a stroke than the general population. Clots can also travel to other parts of the body (kidneys, heart, intestines), causing damage.

Atrial fibrillation can decrease the heart's pumping ability (cardiac output) by as much as 20 to 25 per cent. Therefore this condition, combined with a fast heart rate over a long period of time, can result in heart failure. Chronic atrial fibrillation is associated with an increased risk of death.

Although atrial fibrillation itself isn't usually life-threatening, it is a medical emergency. Treatment includes medication and other interventions in an attempt to alter the heart's electrical system.

Digoxin

Digoxin is a cardiac glycoside extracted from the purple foxglove plant, digitalis. A group of pharmacologically active compounds is extracted from the plant's leaves taken from the second year's growth. Depending on the species, the digitalis plant may contain several deadly physiological and chemically-related cardiac and steroidal glycosides. Thus, digitalis has earned more sinister names: 'Dead Man's Bells' and 'Witches' Gloves'.

The entire plant is toxic (including the roots and seeds), although the leaves of the upper stem are particularly potent, with just a nibble being enough to potentially cause death. Early symptoms of ingestion include nausea, vomiting, diarrhoea, abdominal pain, wild hallucinations, delirium and severe headache. Depending on the severity of the toxicosis the victim may later suffer irregular and slow pulse, tremors, various cerebral disturbances, especially of a visual nature (unusual colour visions with objects appearing yellowish, to green and blue halos around lights), convulsions and deadly disturbances of the heart.

Digoxin is widely used in the treatment of various heart conditions, namely atrial fibrillation, atrial flutter and congestive heart failure that cannot be controlled by other medication. Digoxin preparations are commonly marketed under the trade name Lanoxin. This medicine is highly potent and has a tendency to toxicity in the individual. It is therefore prescribed in micrograms and even then patients may suffer from toxic effects. You may find yourself being asked by a doctor to check digoxin levels in a patient's plasma.

The medicine works in two ways. Firstly, it causes a decrease of conduction of electrical impulses through the AV node. Secondly, it increases the force of contraction via inhibition of what is known as the sodium-potassium pump. This is rather like a revolving door in the wall of a cardiac cell which allows two molecules of potassium into the cell and removes three molecules of sodium. In so doing, it restores the chemical balance between the inside and outside of the cell so that it can contract again.

Digoxin inhibits this 'revolving door' mechanism which results in an increase in the level of sodium ions in the myocytes (cardiac muscle cells). However, the high level of sodium in the myocyte interferes with another 'revolving door'. This door works between sodium and calcium, and its action is slowed down, which means that more calcium is retained by the myocyte. By increasing the amount of calcium in the myocyte, digoxin increases the contractility of the cardiac muscle. It also increases vagal activity via its central action on the central nervous system, thus decreasing the conduction of electrical impulses through the AV node.

Digoxin is usually given by mouth, but can also be given by IV injection in urgent situations (the injection should be delivered slowly with the heart rhythm being monitored). The half-life of the drug is about 36 hours. Digoxin is given once daily, usually in 125 or 250mcg amounts. In patients with decreased kidney function the half-life is considerably longer, calling for a reduction in dosing or a switch to a different glycoside (such as digitoxin, which although having a much longer elimination half-life of around seven days, is mainly eliminated from the body via the liver, and thus not affected by changes in renal function).

Effective plasma levels are fairly well defined, 1–2.6mmol/L. In suspected toxicity or ineffectiveness, digoxin levels should be monitored. Plasma potassium levels also need to be closely controlled as people with low potassium levels are more likely to have adverse effects. This is because digoxin and potassium compete for receptors in cardiac muscle tissue; thus if there is less potassium then more digoxin will bind to receptors, increasing the chance of toxicity.

Verapamil

This medicine belongs to a group of drugs known as *calcium blockers* (also known as *calcium channel antagonists*). Since calcium channels are especially concentrated in the SA and AV nodes, calcium blockers can be used to decrease impulse conduction through the AV node, thus protecting the ventricles from atrial tachyarrhythmias (fast heart rates).

Initially verapamil may be given by an IV route and, as with digoxin, the dose is given slowly. Generally, verapamil is given with heart and blood pressure monitoring over at least a two-minute period (at least three minutes in the elderly). The dosage is based on the patient's age, medical condition, body size and response to therapy.

Clinical tip

It is very important that you check that the patient is not currently taking beta blockers as there is a risk of hypotension (low blood pressure) or, even worse, that the heart will stop (asystole) if verapamil is given in this case.

An oral dose of between 40 and 120mg daily is the commonest from of administration. Verapamil prolongs and intensifies the effects of alcohol in the body, therefore the patient should be advised to either avoid or very carefully limit alcoholic beverages when using this medication. Caution is advised when this drug is used in the elderly. It should be used only when clearly needed during pregnancy, and any patient should discuss the risks and benefits with their doctor. This drug is also excreted into breast milk and a decision should be made whether to stop the drug or avoid breast-feeding.

Clinical tip

Verapamil may cause dizziness and light-headedness especially during the first few days, so it is advisable for patients to avoid activities requiring alertness. It is also important to inform patients that when sitting or lying down they should get up *slowly*, to allow their body to adjust and minimize any dizziness. The patient may also complain of weakness, fatigue, nausea, muscle cramps, headache, flushing or constipation. However, these effects should disappear as the body adjusts to the medication. If side-effects persist the patient should be advised to see their doctor without delay.

Drugs that act on both supraventricular and ventricular arrhythmias

There are many drugs that act on both supraventricular and ventricular arrhythmias. However, it is not the intention of this book to swamp you with information. Therefore we have made a decision to focus on three common drugs that you will come across in this group in your clinical practice.

Sotalol

The 'olol' suffix tells us that this drug comes from a group known as beta blockers. These drugs are used to slow the abnormally fast heart rate in certain arrhythmias, such as atrial fibrillation and atrial flutter. As discussed, these arrhythmias arise from the atrium (upper chambers of the heart) and usually cause the pulse to be rapid and irregular. In addition, beta blockers can prevent certain rhythms altogether, most notably supraventricular tachycardia, an arrhythmia associated with frequent rapid bursts of palpitations. Beta blockers have been shown to prevent arrhythmias that lead to sudden cardiac death. Sometimes, doctors combine beta blockers with other anti-arrhythmics for enhanced effects.

Sotalol is used to help prevent paroxysmal supraventricular arrhythmias. It also suppresses ventricular ectopics (an ectopic heartbeat is an irregularity of the heart rate and heart rhythm involving extra or skipped heartbeats). The medicine also supresses ventricular tachycardia. This drug is unique in that it is the only beta blocker that substantially prolongs the heart contraction. This mechanism is not fully understood but is believed to be due to a slowing down of potassium ions leaving the cardiac muscle cell.

For acute arrhythmias 20–120mg sotalol can be given by IV; however, this needs to take place over a period of 10 minutes and the patient must have cardiac monitoring throughout. This injection can be repeated if necessary after a six-hour interval. More normally the drug is given orally, and initially the dose is 80mg divided into one or two doses in a 24-hour period. The dose may then be increased approximately every three days to a usual dose of 160–320mg daily, in two divided doses.

Although most patients are able to take beta blockers without difficulty, there are a number of side-effects. These drugs should be used cautiously if the patient has asthma, emphysema or other lung diseases because beta blockers can worsen the wheezing or airway obstruction seen in these disorders. There is a group of 'selective' beta blockers available that act on the heart much more strongly than on the lungs and these are useful when mild lung disease is present. Examples include metoprolol, bisoprolol and atenolol. However, sotalol comes under the category of non-cardioselective beta blocker.

A further important side-effect of beta blockers is impotence (or erectile dysfunction) in men. This is a fairly common problem, especially since most men who need beta blockers may already be prone to erectile dysfunction (because of the presence of chronic illnesses such as diabetes, hypertension and atherosclerosis). Beta blockers can also cause blood pressure to become too low, and indeed are used to treat patients suffering from hypertension.

In diabetes, it is possible that a beta blocker could make it harder to notice the symptoms of low blood sugar (see Chapter 8 of *Essentials of Pharmacology for Nurses*). Beta blockers can still be very helpful for diabetics, but doctors recommend careful blood glucose monitoring. Finally, beta blockers may cause what we call 'constitutional symptoms', that is, feelings of fatigue, mild depression or lack of energy.

It is important to inform the patient of the need to discuss any side-effects with their doctor. It is always a case-by-case issue whether the benefits of a medicine outweigh the side-effects or risk.

Amiodarone

Amiodarone is used to correct abnormal rhythms of the heart. Although it has many side-effects, some of which are severe and potentially fatal, it has been successful in treating many arrhythmias where other anti-arrhythmic drugs have failed. Amiodarone is considered a 'broad spectrum' anti-arrhythmic medication, which means it has multiple and complex effects on the electrical activity of the heart which is responsible for the organ's rhythm. Despite its multiple electrophysiological effects, it is generally relegated to a second-line drug because of the high incidence of side-effects and drug interactions. It should only be initiated under specialist supervision.

Amiodarone is sometimes used for 'drug cardioversion' of patients in atrial fibrillation, or more controversially to maintain sinus rhythm after cardioversion (where it is more effective than sotalol or propafenone). These techniques are used to return patients to a normal sinus rhythm. There are two types of cardioversion: drug cardioversion and electrical cardioversion. Drug cardioversion uses type 1 anti-arrhythmic medications such as amiodarone to correct irregular heartbeats to a normal rhythm and to slow an overactive heart. Electrical cardioversion (defibrillation) is the choice of most doctors. This technique delivers an electrical current to the heart through two metal plates (paddles) placed on the chest. The sudden burst of electricity through the heart converts the fibrillation back to normal sinus rhythm. Amiodarone is also used after adrenaline in current advanced life support protocols, in shock refractory pulseless ventricular tachycardia (VT) and ventricular fibrillation (VF).

Amiodarone has a structure similar to thyroxine (one of the major hormones produced by the thyroid gland), with high iodine content. It causes little or no myocardial suppression. Amiodarone is best absorbed with food, and is highly lipid soluble, taking many days to reach a steady state if given orally, as it is taken up and stored in adipose tissue, muscle, liver, lungs and skin – in other words, it has a large volume of distribution. IV amiodarone may work more quickly and is the usual route of administration in the acute hospital setting. This drug takes a very long time to be eliminated from the body, the half-life being 58 days. Electrophysiological studies will not usually be undertaken until amiodarone has been eliminated.

The drug works by slowing the heart rate and AV node conduction. The conduction through the AV node comes about as the drug interferes with movement through calcium channels and beta-receptor blockade. There is a slowing of intracardiac conduction as a result of the drug affecting the movement of sodium. Finally, the drug acts on potassium and sodium channels in the cardiac muscle making it more difficult for contraction to take place. In other words, it makes the heart muscle less 'excitable'.

The dose of amiodarone administered is tailored to the individual and the arrhythmia that is being treated. An oral loading dose is typically 200mg, three times a day for one week, reduced to 200mg twice daily for a further week. A maintanence dose is then prescribed of 200mg daily or the minimum required for controlling the arrhythmia. The IV dose, administered in the coronary care setting initially, consists of 5mg for every kg of body weight, delivered over 20–120 minutes with cardiac monitoring. The drug in this case is administered via what is known as a *central line*. This is a catheter placed into a large vein in the body (e.g. the subclavian vein in the chest). It is used to administer medications or fluids and to obtain blood tests and cardiovascular measurements such as the central venous pressure. Certain medications, such as amiodarone, are preferably given through a central line.

Severe (sometimes fatal) lung or liver problems have infrequently occurred in patients using this drug. It is important that you inform the patient that if they experience any of the following serious side-effects they must seek medical advice as soon as possible: cough, fever, chills, chest pain, difficult or painful breathing, severe stomach pain, fatigue, yellowing eyes or skin, dark urine.

Like other medications used to treat irregular heartbeats, amiodarone can infrequently cause the condition to become worse, and, due to the lingering amount of this drug in the body, heartbeat problems may occur months after the patient has stopped taking the drug. Patients should therefore be advised to seek medical advice if their heart continues to pound, skips a beat, is beating very fast or very slowly, or they feel light-headed or faint.

This drug may also cause serious vision changes such as seeing halos and blurred vision. Very rarely, cases of permanent blindness have been reported. Again, patients should seek medical help if such symptoms present. Due to the iodine content of amiodarone, abnormalities in thyroid function are common. Both under- and overactivity of the thyroid may occur and measurement of free thyroxine (FT4) alone may be unreliable in detecting such problems. Therefore thyroid stimulating hormone levels should be checked every six months.

The pharmokinetics of numerous drugs, including many that are commonly administered to individuals with heart disease, are affected by amiodarone. For example, cyclosporine, flecainide, procainamide, quinidine and simvastatin This is because amiodarone inhibits the action of cytochrome P450, a liver enzyme that helps break down drugs. This means that the drugs take longer to be excreted from the body. As a result the drug could build up to levels that are toxic if given alongside amiodarone.

In particular, doses of digoxin should be halved in individuals taking amiodarone. Amiodarone also potentiates the action of warfarin. Individuals taking both of these medications should have their warfarin dose halved and their anticoagulation status (measured as the prothrombin time (PT) and International Normalized Ratio (INR)) measured more frequently. The effect of amiodarone in the warfarin concentration can be as early as a few days after initiation of treatment, or delayed by a few weeks.

Flecainide

Flecainide acetate is a type of medicine used to regulate the rate and rhythm of the heart. The heart's pumping action is controlled by electrical signals that pass through the heart muscle. The electrical signals cause the two pairs of heart chambers (left and right atria and ventricles) to contract in a regular manner that produces the heartbeat. If the electrical activity in the heart is disturbed for any reason, irregular heartbeats (arrhythmias) of various types can result. These can seriously undermine the pumping action of the heart and result in inefficient blood circulation around the body. Flecainide helps to treat arrhythmias by decreasing the sensitivity of the heart muscle cells to electrical impulses. This slows and regulates the electrical conduction in the heart muscle, which helps to restore disturbances in the heart rhythm. There are several different types of arrhythmia. This medicine may be given in the form of tablets or injection, depending on which type of arrhythmia is being treated.

Flecainide infrequently produces very serious, new and irregular arrhythmias. Therefore, it should be used in carefully selected patients to treat life-threatening irregular heartbeats only. The oral dose will be initiated by the cardiologist and ventricular arrhythmias are initially treated with a dose of 100mg being given twice a day. After a period of three to five days the dose is lowered to the lowest to control the abnormal heart rhythm. Slow IV injection in hospital may be administered but this would only be carried out under cardiac monitoring and with resuscitation equipment at hand.

Drugs that act on ventricular arrhythmias

We will only consider one drug under this heading: lignocaine hydrochloride (see also Chapter 3 of *Essentials of Pharmacology for Nurses*). This drug affects the movement of sodium into cells. It is used intravenously for the treatment of ventricular arrhythmias (for acute myocardial infarction, digitalis poisoning, cardioversion or cardiac catherization). However, a routine prophylactic administration is no longer recommended for acute myocardial infarction because the overall benefit of this measure is not convincing. Usually an IV injection of 100mg is administered over a period of a few minutes. The dose may be less in low-weight patients or those who have poor circulation. Following the initial dose the cardiologist will commence the patient on a slow IV regimen in order to control the life-threatening arrhythmias.

Drugs used in cardiac resuscitation

Cardiac arrest is the cessation of normal circulation of the blood due to failure of the heart to contract effectively, and if this is unexpected can be termed a sudden cardiac arrest. In adults, sudden cardiac arrest results primarily from cardiac disease (of all types, but especially coronary artery disease). In a significant percentage of people, sudden cardiac arrest is the first manifestation of heart disease. Other causes include circulatory shock from non-cardiac disorders (especially pulmonary embolism, GI haemorrhage and trauma), respiratory failure and metabolic disturbance (including drug overdose).

In children, cardiac causes of sudden cardiac arrest are much less common. Instead, predominant causes include trauma, poisoning and various respiratory problems (e.g. airway obstruction, smoke inhalation, drowning, infection and sudden infant death syndrome).

Only a small number of drugs are indicated during cardiac arrest and we have already discussed two that can be used – adenosine and amiodarone. Two further drugs will be considered in this section: adrenaline and atropine.

Adrenaline

Adrenaline is a natural stimulant made in the adrenal glands, which lie just above the kidneys. It is carried in the bloodstream and affects the autonomic nervous system, which controls functions such as the heart rate. Adrenaline is the body's activator, and is released in response to anxiety,

exercise or fear. This is the basis of the so-called 'fight-or-flight' reaction. When an individual is threatened, the options are usually either to stand and fight or to run away as fast as possible. Both responses require extra supplies of blood and oxygen in the muscles. Fright causes the brain to send signals to the adrenal glands which start pumping large amounts of adrenaline into the bloodstream. This increases the heart and breathing rates in preparation for the ensuing action.

The effects of adrenaline are harnessed in a cardiac arrest situation and it is the first drug given in all causes of cardiac arrest. Adrenaline concentrates the blood around the vital organs, specifically the brain and the heart, by peripheral vasoconstriction. These are the organs that must continue to receive blood to increase the chances of survival following cardiac arrest. Adrenaline also strengthens cardiac contractions as it stimulates the cardiac muscle. This further increases the amount of blood circulating to the vital organs, and also increases the chance of the heart returning to a normal rhythm.

Adrenaline can be given repeatedly during a cardiac arrest until the condition of the patient improves. The Resuscitation Council recommends that it is given as soon as possible after a cardiac arrest has been identified. This can be repeated every three to five minutes. Even though in a cardiac arrest situation care is being administered rapidly, it is still vital to document the time, route and amount of adrenaline being administered.

The suggested administration route is by central line, as this allows the drug to reach the cardiac tissue more rapidly. If this is not available, adrenaline may be administered through a cannula in a peripheral vein.

> ## Clinical tip
>
> If adrenaline is administered through a cannula, the cannula should be flushed with at least 20ml of 0.9 per cent sodium chloride after the drug has been given. This will ensure the entry of the drug into the circulation.

Manufacturers suggest that adrenaline may be injected directly into the heart through the chest wall if no other route is available. This can be a difficult procedure and should only be attempted by a competent clinician and when all other attempts to gain access have failed.

Once an organized rhythm has been established the use of adrenaline must be reassessed, as excess amounts can cause the patient to develop ventricular fibrillation. It is also important to understand that adrenaline reacts with sodium bicarbonate to produce solid material. For this reason these two drugs should not be administered through the same IV route without adequate flushing with 0.9 per cent sodium chloride.

Atropine

The vagus nerve is part of the parasympathetic nervous system which in turn is part of the autonomic nervous system. However, unlike the action of the fight-or-flight system the parasympathetic system is resonsible for *slowing* the heart. The drug atropine blocks the actions of the vagus nerve on the heart, making it useful when a patient has a very slow heart rate (bradycardia). Blocking the vagus activity should help to speed up the cardiac rate.

This drug should be administered intravenously and the dose depends on the heart rhythm. For bradycardia a dose of 0.5mg should be given and repeated every five minutes until a satisfactory heart rate is achieved. Atropine is no longer recommended for routine use in asystole or pulseless electrical activity.

Wolff-Parkinson-White syndrome

Wolff-Parkinson-White syndrome involves episodes of rapid heart rate (tachycardia) caused by abnormal electrical pathways (circuits) in the heart, which are often present from birth. It is also sometimes referred to in textbooks as 'pre-excitation syndrome'. A 'syndrome' is simply a collection of symptoms described by the patient.

As described earlier in this chapter, normally the electrical stimulus of the heart travels through the upper chambers (atria) and then through the AV node where it is delayed before continuing into the lower chambers or ventricles. In Wolff-Parkinson-White syndrome there is an 'accessory' or extra AV conduction pathway which bypasses the normal conduction delay of the AV node and causes a rapid heart rate to be initiated in the upper chambers (a supraventricular tachycardia), called a re-entry tachycardia. An atrioventricular re-entrant tachycardia occurs when this system of cardiac conduction is short-circuited in a way that allows an impulse to create a self-perpetuating and uncontrolled fast heart rhythm. If the rate is too fast, its efficiency falls and symptoms such as blackouts, fainting, chest tightness or shortness of breath can result. The extra pathway in Wolff-Parkinson-White syndrome can often be located very precisely.

Wolff-Parkinson-White syndrome occurs in around 4 in 100,000 people, and is one of the most common causes of fast heart rate disorder in young children and adolescents. The person concerned may be totally unaware of the condition, or symptoms may include palpitations (sensation of feeling heart beat), dizziness, light-headedness or fainting. There may also be chest pain, tightness or breathlessness.

Examination during an episode of palpitation usually reveals a pulse rate of 150 per minute in the presence of a normal or low blood pressure. Investigations can include ECG and continuous ambulatory ECG monitoring in an attempt to demonstrate diagnostic findings. Medications may be used to control or prevent rapid heartbeat. These include adenosine, anti-arrhythmics and amiodarone.

Case studies

① Mrs Walker is a 72-year-old woman who has been admitted to the medical unit following a general deterioration in her health and ability to carry out most of the activities of living independently.

She doesn't think through daily problems as quickly as before, she makes mistakes balancing her cheque book, she is more sedentary, fatigues easily and is winded when carrying her shopping. On examination she has oedema, her blood pressure is 160/90, her pulse is 88 beats per minute and her weight is 75kg. Her current medications are glipizide (2.5mg daily), lisinopril (20mg daily), atorvastatin (40mg daily), aspirin (75mg daily), felodipine (5mg daily) and hydrochlorothiazide (25mg daily).

■ Her daughter approaches you for information regarding atorvastatin. What responses would you give?

② Four years ago, when he was in his late fifties, Geoff began to feel breathless and tight-chested on his daily walk to work. 'It was just over a mile and I enjoyed the exercise, particularly in the nicer weather, but in the spring I just wasn't feeling right,' he remembers. After a few days of discomfort, which wore off as soon as he sat down at his desk in the council offices where he worked, Geoff decided to see his doctor. 'I actually thought I had a chest infection,' he says. He was immediately started on daily aspirin treatment to thin his blood and prevent him having a heart attack if a blood clot got caught in the most narrowed coronary artery. 'I was also given a drug called glyceryl trinitrate, which is delivered by spraying it into your mouth, like a breath freshener,' says Geoff.

■ Geoff wants you to recap how his GTN is helping him. What would you say?

Key learning points

Introduction

➢ Cardiovascular disease costs the NHS in the UK nearly £15 billion annually.

Atherosclerosis

➢ Atherosclerosis is a degenerative disease that results in narrowing of the arteries.

Cholesterol

➢ Cholesterol itself is not harmful, but high blood cholesterol can be dangerous.

Normal cholesterol level

➢ The DH recommends that cholesterol levels should be less than 5mmol/L.

Lipid regulating drugs

➢ Lowering the amount of low-density lipoproteins and raising the levels of high-density lipoproteins slows the progression of atherosclerosis and may even cause a reduction in its formation.

Statins

➢ Statins block the enzyme in the liver that is responsible for making cholesterol.

←

Fibrates

➢ Fibrates lower blood triglyceride levels by reducing the liver's production of VLDLs and by speeding up the removal of triglycerides from the blood.

Bile-acid binding resins

➢ Bile-acid binding resins work by binding to bile in the digestive tract.

Angina

➢ This is chest discomfort that occurs when there is a decreased blood oxygen supply to an area of the heart muscle.

Glyceryl trinitrate

➢ Belongs to a group of drugs called nitrates that contain the chemical nitric oxide and has the effect of making the veins and arteries relax and widen (dilate).

Isosorbide mononitrate and dinitrate

➢ These drugs will not be effective in a person who is having an angina attack.

Electrical conduction through the heart

➢ The normal heart begins with an electrical impulse from the SA node, located high in the right atrium.

Contraction of cardiac muscle

➢ In order for the myocardium to contract, sodium must enter the muscle cell.

Paroxysmal supraventricular tyachycardia

➢ A regular, fast heart rate that begins and ends suddenly and originates in heart tissue other than that in the ventricles.

Adenosine

➢ Slows down the electrical impulses through the atrioventricular node.

Atrial fibrillation

➢ An irregular and often rapid heart rate that commonly causes poor blood flow to the body and symptoms of heart palpitations, shortness of breath and weakness.

Digoxin

➢ Increases the force of contraction via inhibition of the sodium-potassium pump.

→

←

Verapamil

➤ Belongs to a group of drugs called calcium blockers (calcium channel antagonists).

Sotalol

➤ Comes from a group of drugs known as beta blockers and is used to help prevent paroxysmal supraventricular arrhythmias, ventricular ectopics and ventricular tachycardia.

Amiodarone

➤ Considered a 'broad spectrum' anti-arrhythmic medication.

Flecainide

➤ Helps to treat arrhythmias by decreasing the sensitivity of the heart muscle cells to electrical impulses.

Drugs that act on ventricular arrhythmias

➤ Lignocaine is used intravenously for the treatment of ventricular arrhythmias.

Adrenaline

➤ The first drug given in all causes of cardiac arrest.

Atropine

➤ Blocks the actions of the vagus nerve on the heart.

Wolff-Parkinson-White syndrome

➤ Involves episodes of rapid heart rate (tachycardia) caused by abnormal electrical pathways (circuits) in the heart, which are often present from birth.

Calculations

1 A patient is ordered 30mg of Diltiazem hydrochloride. 60mg tablets are available. How many tablets will you give?

2 A doctor has prescribed 0.25mg of digoxin. You have 125mcg tablets in stock. How many should you give?

3 A doctor has prescribed a patient 125mcg of digoxin. You have digoxin elixir 50mcg per ml. How much should you administer?

4   A patient with cardiovascular disease is taking six tablets per day. How many will they take in a week?

5   How many ml of digoxin liquid containing 50mcg/ml are required to give a dose of 62.5mcg?

6   An infusion pump contains 50mg of glyceryl trinitrate in 100ml. You are asked to deliver a dose of 4mg per hour. What is the rate in ml per hour?

7   You are required to give a patient GTN as a continuous IV infusion at 25mcg/minute. You have prepared a 50mg in 50ml infusion. What rate should you set the infusion pump at, in ml/hr, to deliver this dose?

8   A patient is prescribed an amiodarone infusion of 400mg in 200ml and the flow rate is 35ml/hr. What would the hourly dose be?

9   A patient on the cardiovascular ward is receiving an IV infusion. The patient is to receive 1L of fluid over the next five hours. What volume of fluid (in ml) will they receive each hour?

10   Digoxin elixir contains 50mcg in 1ml. How much would you need to give a dose of 0.1mg?

For further assistance with calculations, please see Meriel Hutton's book *Essential Calculation Skills for Nurses, Midwives and Healthcare Practitioners* (Open University Press 2009).

Multiple choice questions

1 The government recommends that cholesterol levels should be:

a) 5mmol/L
b) Less than 5mmol/L
c) More than 5mmol/L
d) Dependent on the individual

2 Statins work by

a) Raising the metabolic rate
b) Blocking the absorption of cholesterol
c) Blocking the production of bile
d) Blocking the enzyme in the liver that is responsible for making cholesterol

3 Fibrates reduce the liver's production of

a) Very low density lipoproteins
b) Low-density lipoproteins
c) High-density lipoproteins
d) All of the above

4 Colesevelam is an example of

a) A bile-acid binding resin
b) A statin
c) A fibrate
d) A nitrate

→

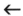

5 Glyceryl trinitrate is not administered orally because

a) The drug molecule is too big to be absorbed by the body
b) Stomach acid destroys the drug
c) It has a bad taste
d) Most of the drug is destroyed by the first pass effect

6 Digoxin is given daily as its half-life is

a) 4 hours
b) 16 hours
c) 36 hours
d) 8 hours

7 Which of the following drugs is a calcium channel blocker?

a) Digoxin
b) Verapamil
c) Isosorbide mononitrate
d) Amiodarone

8 Amiodarone has a high

a) Sodium content
b) Magnesium content
c) Calcium content
d) Iodine content

9 Lignocaine is used to treat

a) Both supra and ventricular arrhythmias
b) Supra-ventricular arrhythmias
c) Ventricular arrhythmias
d) Heart block

10 In cardiac arrest atropine is given because

a) It is naturally occurring
b) It stimulates parasympathetic activity
c) It is a more potent drug than adrenaline
d) Blocking vagus activity could help speed up cardiac rate

Recommended further reading

Barber, P. and Robertson, D. (2012) *Essentials of Pharmacology for Nurses*, 2nd edn. Maidenhead: Open University Press.

Beckwith, S. and Franklin, P. (2007) *Oxford Handbook of Nurse Prescribing*. Oxford: Oxford University Press.

Brenner, G.M. and Stevens, C.W. (2006) *Pharmacology*, 2nd edn. Philadelphia, PA: Saunders Elsevier.

British Heart Foundation (2011) *Coronary Heart Disease Statistics in UK, February 2011*. London: British Heart Foundation.

Clayton, B.D. (2009) *Basic Pharmacology for Nurses*, 14th edn. St Louis, MO: Mosby Elsevier.

Coben, D. and Atere-Roberts, E. (2005) *Calculations for Nursing and Healthcare*, 2nd edn. Basingstoke: Palgrave Macmillan.

Conway, B. and Fuat, A. (2007) Recent advances in angina management: implications for nurses, *Nursing Standard*, 21(38): 49.

Downie, G., Mackenzie, J. and Williams, A. (2007) *Pharmacology and Medicines Management for Nurses*, 4th edn. Edinburgh: Churchill Livingstone.

Gallimore, D. (2006) Understanding the drugs used during cardiac arrest response, *Nursing Times*, 102(23): 24–6.

Gatford, J.D. and Phillips, N. (2006) *Nursing Calculations*, 7th edn. Edinburgh: Churchill Livingstone Elsevier.

Hutton, M. (2009) *Essential Calculation Skills for Nurses, Midwives and Healthcare Practitioners*. Maidenhead: Open University Press.

Karch, A.M. (2008) *Focus on Nursing Pharmacology*, 4th edn. Philadelphia, PA: Lippincott Williams & Wilkins.

NICE (National Institute for Health and Clinical Excellence) (2008) *Technology Appraisal 094: Statins for the Prevention of Cardiovascular Events*. London: NICE.

Senior, K. (2010) *Facts and Figures: Heart Disease in the UK*, www.cardiacmatters.co.uk/facts-figures-heart-disease-uk.html.

Simonson, T., Aarbakke, J., Kay, I., Coleman, I., Sinnott, P. and Lyssa, R. (2006) *Illustrated Pharmacology for Nurses*. London: Hodder Arnold.

Starkings, S. and Krause, L. (2010) *Passing Calculation Tests for Nursing Students*. Exeter: Learning Matters.

Turner, A. and Jowett, N. (2006) NT clinical: the role of statin therapy in preventing recurrent stroke, *Nursing Times*, 102(38): 25–6.

Drugs acting on the gastrointestinal tract

2

Chapter contents

Learning objectives

After studying this chapter you should be able to:

- Briefly explain the epidemiology and aetiology of gastrointestinal disease.
- Demonstrate a basic understanding of how gastric secretions are involved in the breakdown of foodstuffs in the stomach.
- Describe what is meant by a gastrointestinal disorder.
- Demonstrate an awareness of the role of natural painkillers within the body (prostaglandins).
- Review the physiology of carbohydrate and protein synthesis.
- Compare and contrast the modes of action between different drug classifications used in the treatment of gastrointestinal disorders.
- Use basic maths to calculate simple drug dosages.

Introduction

The gastrointestinal (GI) tract, also known as the *digestive* or *alimentary tract*, forms a continuous tube from the mouth to the rectum which is open at both ends. It measures about 10 metres from opening to opening and is designed to deliver food and nutrients to the appropriate organs of the body for digestion, absorption and utilization.

Along with oxygen, food and water are vital elements to the survival of life. Without them every cell in the body would eventually starve and die, resulting in possible multi-organ failure and consequently death. The energy derived from food and water is utilized by the body to form new cells and repair damaged tissue.

There are five basic activities carried out by the GI tract:

1. **Ingestion:** taking food into the mouth. *Mastication* is the term used for the chewing, biting and grinding of food while in the mouth.
2. **Peristalsis:** the movement by which food is propelled along the alimentary tract.
3. **Digestion:** the process by which food is rendered absorbable.
4. **Absorption:** the process of absorbing nutrients from the GI tract for distribution to the body cells and structures.
5. **Elimination:** the passage of waste from the body via urine and faeces.

Ingestion

The oral cavity (mouth) is the first location that food usually enters the body. Along with the teeth and tongue, which aid in the chewing and grinding of food into manageable pieces to be swallowed, three pairs of salivary glands (parotid, submandibular and sublingual) begin the process of producing saliva, which is brought about by the presence of food in the mouth or by a learned or conditioned reflex that starts saliva production resulting from the sight, smell or thought of food. As saliva is made up of 90–95 per cent water, this moistens the food bolus which is moved around the mouth by the tongue and chewed with the teeth (mastication). The pH of saliva is 7–8 which makes it alkilitic in nature (no acid). The amount of saliva produced varies throughout the day, but on average a person produces approximately 1–1.5L/day. The main constituent of saliva is a ferment called ptyalin (salivary amylase) which begins the chemical breakdown of starch into sugar. As the food is swallowed, the action of ptyalin continues this process for about 20 minutes once food passes into the stomach, until it is rendered acidic by the action of gastric fluid. Protein digestion does not begin in the mouth owing to the pH of saliva. Many nutritionists, however, believe that the first stage of digestion begins in the mouth as a result of adequate chewing and moistioning of food into manageable amounts to be swallowed; this in turn aids the breakdown of food *before* reaching the stomach.

Peristalsis

Peristalsis is described as the successive waves of involuntary contractions that pass along the wall of a hollow muscular structure, like the oesophagus or intestines. This process is under the control of the medulla of the brainstem which starts the first part of swallowing by parasympathetic motor impulses (facial nerve, vagus nerve, mesenteric plexus). After food has been chewed into a bolus, it is swallowed and moved towards the back of the mouth into the pharynx where the soft palate shuts off the nasopharynx, prohibiting food entering the nasal cavity. The glottis closes by muscular contraction while the constrictor muscles of the pharynx take hold of the bolus of food and pass it into the oesophagus. When this action is coordinated properly the trachea is bypassed and food is not able to enter it.

The oesophagus itself has four layers of tissue: a fibrous outer layer, a muscular layer (which has both longitudinal and circular fibres), a submucous layer (containing large blood vessels and nerves) and an inner mucous membrane that secretes mucous to moisten the surface of the oesophagus which helps to minimize friction when swallowing. As food passes into the oesophagus, circular muscle fibres contract immediately behind the bolus which constricts the oesophagus and forces the bolus downwards. The longitutinal fibres of the musclar coating immediately in front of the bolus simultaneously contract, shortening and expanding this section of the oesophagus. Ultimately these 'waves of dilation' followed by 'waves of contraction' produce the peristaltic movement to shift the bolus of food towards the cardiac sphincter at the entrance of the stomach. If food is chewed properly in the mouth and coated with enough lubricant this action should be unimpeded. However, sometimes the bolus of food is poorly lubricated and, when this happens, stretch receptors in the oesophageal lining are stimulated and a local reflex response causes a secondary peristaltic wave around the bolus which forces it further down the oesophagus. The secondary wave will continue until the bolus enters the stomach. This process can often be felt by the patient as having something stuck in the oesophagus or having difficulty swallowing. A drink will sometimes aid the movement of the bolus.

The speed of swallowing is determined by the consistency of the food or liquid that has been ingested and whether the person is sitting or standing. Allowing for these factors, on average a bolus of food or fluid can take between 1 and 8 seconds to reach the cardiac sphincter.

> ### Clinical tip
>
>
> A side-effect of certain drugs used to treat illnesses such as depression, anxiety, pain, allergies, congestion and diarrhoea is 'dry mouth' which affects the lubrication of food in the mouth and oesophagus.

Digestion

There are three mechanical tasks that the stomach is responsible for. Firstly, as it is the most dilated part of the digestive tract, it has the ability to store swallowed food and liquids. The upper part of the stomach relaxes to accept large volumes of swallowed material (approximately 1500ml in an adult). The inner layer of the stomach is a honeycombed mucous membrane that has numerous folds called *rugae*, which run longitudinally and flatten out when the stomach is full. This membrane is responsible for continuing the process of lubrication by the presence of goblet cells which produce mucous. Next, food is mixed with digestive juices (pepsinogen, hydrochloric acid, intrinsic factor and gastrin) that are produced by the stomach, the lower part of the stomach mixing these materials by muscular action. The third task is to empty the stomach contents slowly into the first part of the small intestine (duodenum).

There are a number of factors that affect the emptying of the stomach, including the kind of food ingested and the degree of muscle action needed for the churning and breaking down of foodstuffs. Liquids remain in the stomach for about 30 minutes, and solid foods remain for approximately two to four hours. Carbohydrates (bread and starches) spend the least amount of time in the stomach, whereas protein remains there for longer, and fats in general, the longest. The breakdown of all foodstuffs eventually produces a semi-fluid mass of partly digested food called *chyme*, which is slowly expelled into the duodenum where the extraction of nutrients begins.

Absorption

Chyme entering the duodenum is very acidic with a pH of about 2. To raise its pH, the duodenum secretes a hormone called cholecystokinin (CCK) which causes the gall bladder to contract, releasing alkaline bile into the duodenum. Another hormone, called *secretin*, stimulates a large amount of sodium bicarbonate, which raises the chyme's pH to 7 before it reaches the jejunum. As the pH is now 7 the enzymes that were present in the stomach are no longer active and this leads to a further breakdown of the nutrients still present by anaerobic bacteria. These bacteria help to synthesize vitamin B and vitamin K.

As chyme passes through the duodenum into the upper part of the small intestine its focus remains upon digestion and absorption, with most of the digested molecules of food being absorbed within the small intestine. The mucosa of the small intestine contains a number of folds that are covered with finger-like projections called *villi*. These are covered with microscopic projections called *microvilli*. These structures create a vast surface area through which nutrients can be absorbed into the bloodstream to other parts of the body for storage or further chemical alteration.

Elimination

After the intense activity within the small intestine, where most digestion has taken place, the large intestine consists mainly of water, salts and cellulose (which is indigestible), along with bacteria. Very little food material is left. Although the bacteria are largely killed in the stomach by the high acid content, the warm, moist alkaline environment of the large intestine encourages the growth of any remaining bacteria. As the material within the large colon is in a very fluid state, the transverse colon's role is to reabsorb fluid back into the body. This in turn rapidly makes the remaining fluid into a paste containing the cellulose and bacteria, and, because of the reabsorbtion of the water, many of the bacteria die. This paste forms the faeces and roughly consists of 50 per cent cellulose and 50 per cent dead bacteria. Peristalsis within the large intestine occurs three to four times a day, moving the faeces into the descending colon. Defaecation (bowel movement) occurs when the movement of the faeces causes the rectum to distend and expel its content.

Helicobacter pylori

Helicobacter pylori (HP) is a gram negative micro-aerophilic (i.e. it requires oxygen to survive), corkscrew-shaped bacterium with the ability to change shape and adapt to its surroundings so that it is able inhabit various areas of the stomach and duodenum. In its spiral guise it has four to six flagella (tail-like projections from the cell body of certain prokaryotic and eukaryotic cells) that allow it motility. Once settled in the stomach lining it changes shape to a coccoid (spherical) form.

HP has a unique way of adapting to the harsh acidic environment of the stomach and causes a low level of inflammation of the stomach lining. It has been identified as contributing to the development of duodenal and gastric ulcers. Ironically, over 80 per cent of infected individuals remain symptom free. Ultimately there appears to be strong evidence for its role in the development of stomach cancer.

Over 50 per cent of the world's population, that is to say, about 3 billion people, harbour the HP bacterium in the upper GI tract. The infection rate has been noted to be higher in developing countries and diminishing in western countries. There is little known about the actual route of transmission, although there is a high incidence of individuals being infected in childhood. One possible explanation is that HP may be transmitted orally by means of faecal matter via tainted food or water. Therefore clean drinking water and hand hygiene are paramount in slowing down the spread of the bacterium.

Pathophysiology

The inside of the stomach produces and is bathed in about 2–3 litres of gastric juice every day. One of the major properties of gastric juice is hydrochloric acid made by the parietal cells in the stomach, the main action of which is to tear apart the toughest foodstuffs and destroy any micro-organisms that are ingested on or within those foodstuffs. The stomach is protected from its own gastric juices by a thick layer of mucous that covers the lining of the stomach and it is in this lining that HP takes advantage of the safe environment of the higher pH and survives. Once established, HP is able to fight the stomach acid that does reach it with its own enzyme called *urease*. Urease converts urea (nitrogenous end product of protein metabolism, of which there is an abundant supply in the stomach from gastric juices and saliva) into bicarbonate and ammonia, which are strong bases. This creation of acid in neutralizing chemicals around the bacterium ultimately protects it from the acid in the stomach.

Clinical tip

The reaction of urea hydrolysis is important for the diagnosis of HP using a breath test.

It was considered once that the stomach was a sterile environment and did not contain any bacteria. Because the stomach has such a low pH of stomach acid (1–4) it was considered that nothing would, or could, survive such a hostile environment; however, the identification and isolation of HP 25 years ago changed this way of thinking.

In reaction to the presence of HP the body's natural defences are activated despite not being able to reach the bacterium in the stomach lining. About 70 per cent of the body's immune system is found in the digestive tract and is often referred to as *gut-associated lymphoid tissue* (GALT) which is an example of mucosa-associated lymphoid tissue. The immune system responds by sending the relevant killer T and B cells, but these cells do not reach their target to eradicate it. Thus the immune system continues to respond, increasing the overall immune response. The breakdown of some T and B cells creates polymorphs, and as they are destroyed they release superoxide radicals onto the cell lining of the stomach. As the immune system sends extra nutrients to reinforce the white cells, HP, as an opportunist, uses these to feed upon. This inflammatory response is called *gastritis* and may potentially lead to a peptic ulcer. The condition is therefore not a *direct* result of HP bacterium but of the inflammation of the stomach lining in response to the bacterium. The type of ulcer that develops depends upon the location of the gastritis, which occurs at the site of HP colonization.

Diagnosis

Diagnosis of the infection is usually made by checking for dyspeptic symptoms. As indicated in the clinical tip above, one non-invasive test is to request patients to drink C or C-labelled urea, which HP metabolizes, producing labelled carbon dioxide which can be detected on the breath. The most reliable method, however, is a biopsy with a rapid urease test, histological exam and microbial culture. Once HP is detected treatment can begin.

Treatment

The standard first-line treatment for HP infection is to eradicate the bacteria and allow any ulcers heal. The treatment consists of a one-week 'triple therapy' consisting of a proton pump inhibitor (PPI) such as omeprazole and two types of antibiotic such as clarithromycin and amoxicillin.

As noted above, HP has been indicated as a potential risk for developing stomach cancer (gastric adenocarcinomas – 70–90 per cent), with its presence having a sixfold risk for gastric cancer. This accounts for about half of all gastric cancers. This has led pathologists to believe that chronic gastritis leads to internal metaplasia (cell changes) which then become malignant.

Drugs that inhibit/neutralize acid

Proton pump inhibitors

PPIs are one the most frequently prescribed classes of drug worldwide, due to their efficiency and low toxicity. However, there is evidence to suggest that PPIs are over-prescribed and that between 25 and 70 per cent of patients have no real indication of needing them. This has had an adverse affect on the National Health Service (NHS) budget, with approximately £100 million being spent unnecessarily. The National Institute for Health and Clinical Excellence (NICE) recommends that PPIs should only be prescribed for actual symptoms of acid reflux, and not as a prophylactic treatment, as is the case for some patients.

Although H2 receptor antagonists such as ranitidine (which can be bought over the counter) are just as effective, and less expensive, the prescribed use of PPIs is astonishing, and they account for over 90 per cent of the NHS drug budget for treating dyspepsia.

Although the efficacy of PPIs in short-term management of gastric acidity has the greatest benefit to patients, their long-term use is not without health risks in some groups. Taking PPIs has the potential to cause an increase in the prevalence of pneumonia and *Campylobacter enteritis* as well as doubling the risk of infection from *Clostridium difficile*. They have also been implicated in the increased rate of hip fractures, possibly due to altered calcium absorption. There may also be (unproven yet possible) altered vitamin B12 and iron absorption related to the alteration of the gastric pH. Rarer conditions such as nephritis and osteoporosis have also been documented.

PPIs include omeprazole, lansoprazole, pantroprazole and rabeprazole. They work by inhibiting gastric acid by blocking the H+/K+ adenosine triphosphate (ATP) enzyme system (the proton pump) of the gastric parietal cell.

Omeprazole

Omeprazole was the first generic PPI to be introduced, in 2002, and now comprises more than four-fifths of all prescribed PPIs in the UK. It has been used successfully to treat duodenal ulcers, gastric ulcers and oesophagitis and may also have a place in the prevention of stress ulceration in the acutely ill and in burns patients. With each of these conditions omeprazole is used in various strengths over various time frames for full effectiveness.

This drug undergoes rapid and almost complete metabolism and no unchanged drug is excreted in the urine. However, approximately 20 per cent of the unchanged drug may be recovered in the faeces. Clearance of omeprazole is not influenced by any renal disease or by haemodialysis. Omeprazole degrades in the presence of moisture, so to prevent degradation by gastric acid the granules in each capsule are enteric-coated.

> ### Clinical tip
>
> Omeprazole inhibits cytochrome P drug metabolism and therefore enhances the effects of warfarin, phenytoin and diazepam.

Cimetidine

This drug is classed as an H2 receptor (histamine receptor) antagonist whose action is to reduce the secretion of gastric acid and pepsin (an enzyme which helps the digestion of protein). The action of histamine in the stomach is to bind to H2 receptor sites and stimulate acid-producing cells on the stomach wall to release acid. Cimetidine works by occupying H2-receptor sites, preventing histamine from triggering the production of acid. This reduction of acid and pepsin allows the healing of ulcers in the stomach and in the duodenum. Cimetidine is also used in the treatment of acid reflux and oesophagitis. The general term which describes this range of symptoms is gastro-oesophageal reflux disease (GORD). Some of the symptoms of GORD (with or without oesophagitis) include heartburn (although this has nothing to do directly with the heart), pain in the upper abdomen and chest, sickness, bloating and belching. A common symptom is a burning pain when swallowing a hot drink.

Prostaglandins

Prostaglandins are a large group of lipid compounds derived from fatty acids which are produced by body tissues. They are mediators that have physiological effects such as smooth muscle contraction, inflammation, gastric secretion and blood clotting. Cyclo-oxygenase 1 (COX1) is an enzyme which produces prostaglandins (natural painkillers) in the stomach. They work by amplifying the electrical signal coming from the nerves which increases the pain that is felt. The role of prostaglandins in the stomach is to maintain blood flow and protect the stomach lining from the corrosive effects of stomach acid. When an ulcer develops in the stomach, prostaglandins produce pain and inflammation at the site of the damaged tissue.

Non-steroidal anti-inflammatory drugs (NSAIDs) like aspirin and ibuprofen block the action of the COX1 enzyme along with another enzyme known as COX2, which is responsible for inflammation in other areas of the body, but not found in the stomach. When the COX1 enzyme is blocked, inflammation is reduced, but the protective mucous lining of the stomach is also reduced which may lead to ulceration and bleeding from the stomach and intestines. Drugs that selectively block COX2 enzymes do not present the same risk of injuring the stomach or intestines. However, they are more likely to cause side-effects on the heart than traditional NSAIDs. This makes them less suitable for patients with heart or circulation problems.

Misoprostol

Misoprostol is a prostaglandin which causes contraction of the smooth muscle in the GI tract and uterus. It is responsible for the dilation of blood vessels and therefore should not be taken during pregnancy as doing so can cause spontaneous abortion. As it also dilates blood vessels it can cause hypotension (low blood pressure), especially in older patients. The action of misoprostol is to reduce the amount of acid that is secreted in the stomach. It is used to promote the healing of gastric and duodenal ulcers.

Drugs that protect the mucosa of the stomach

These drugs that are considered to be *cytoprotective*, meaning that they form a protective barrier over the surface of an ulcer.

Bismuth chelate

Bismuth chelate's actions are to help to protect the gastric mucosa by inhibiting the action of pepsin, promoting synthesis of protective prostaglandins while stimulating the secretion of bicarbonate, which helps to neutralize acid. Bismuth also kills bacteria which are believed to contribute to the aggravation of duodenal ulcers. Unwanted side-effects include nausea, vomiting and blackening of the tongue and faeces. Bismuth is potentially neurotoxic.

Sucralfate

Sucralfate is thought to act by protecting the mucosa from acid-pepsin attack in gastritis and the consequent development of duodenal ulcers. In an acidic environment it forms a gel with mucous and binds to the ulcer base to form a protective barrier to acid and pepsin. It is not absorbed, however, and 30 per cent of the drug can be still found in the stomach three hours after taking it.

Clinical tip

Do not give antacids with sucralfate as they will reduce the effect. Should an antacid be needed, it should not be taken half an hour before or after taking sucralfate. Be aware that sucralfate also reduces the absorption of some antibiotics, theophylline, tetracycline, digoxin and amitriptyline. It also reduced the effectiveness of phenytoin, warfarin and digoxin.

Irritable bowel syndrome

Irritable bowel syndrome (IBS) is a functional bowel disorder characterized by chronic abdominal pain, discomfort, bloating and alteration of bowel habits, in the absence of any detectable organic causes. IBS may alternate between diarrhoea and constipation. It has been estimated by gastroenterologists that as many as one in five adults in the UK suffers from IBS at any one time and of these adults 13 per cent are women and 5 per cent are men. Although there is no cure for IBS there are recommended treatments that aim to relieve symptoms. These include dietary adjustments, medication and patient education. Although distressing, IBS never leads to bowel cancer or permanent bowel damage.

IBS can be classified under four headings:

- diarrhoea-predominant (IBS-D);
- constipation-predominant (IBS-C);
- IBS with alternating stool pattern (IBS-A);
- post-infectious (IBS-PI) – this type of IBS is usually acute onset, develops after an infectious illness and is usually characterized by two or more of the following: fever, vomiting, diarrhoea or a positive stool culture.

Diet

Many different dietary modifications have been attempted to improve the symptoms of IBS. As lactose intolerance and IBS have similar symptoms, patients are often advised to trial a lactose-free diet. While many patients believe they have some form of dietary intolerance, evidence has been disappointing in determining food sensitivities in most patients.

Drugs affecting gut motility

Loperamide

Loperamide is an anti-diarrhoeal drug that works by acting on opioid receptors that are found in the muscle lining the walls of the intestines. By acting on these receptor sites loperamide reduces the muscular contractions of the intestine and slows down peristalsis (the worm-like movement which propels the contents of food and faecal matter through the gut). As the speed of peristalsis is reduced there is more time for water and electrolytes to be reabsorbed from the gut back into the body. This has the effect of firmer stools being formed which are passed less frequently.

Codeine phosphate

Codeine phosphate is a weak opioid (producing morphine-like effects) analgesic that has a role in the management of uncomplicated acute diarrhoea in adults. It activates opioid receptor sites found on the smooth muscles of the bowel which in turn reduces peristalsis and delays the passage of faeces, allowing more water to be absorbed by the large colon. If pain accompanies diarrhoea then codeine phosphate also acts as pain relief. Dependence on this particular drug can develop over a period of time.

Antispasmodics

Mebeverine

Mebeverine is a musculotropic antispasmodic drug that is a direct relaxant of smooth muscle which is beneficial in IBS and diverticular disease. It works by acting directly on the smooth muscle in the gut, causing it to relax. This relieves painful muscle spasms of the gut without affecting its normal motility.

The tablet is taken three times a day, preferably 20 minutes before meals, as this will help relieve symptoms that are worse after eating. When symptoms have improved, usually after several weeks, the dose can be gradually reduced.

Hyoscine (Baclofen)

The action of this drug is to reduce intestinal motility by decreasing the effects of the parasympathetic transmitter acetylcholine (which promotes peristalsis in the GI tract), on the smooth muscles of the intestines. Patients taking medications for high blood pressure (antihypertensive) need to be aware that this drug can increase the blood-pressure-lowering effects which may in turn lead to hypotension (low blood pressure).

Drugs used in inflammatory bowel disorders

Inflammatory bowel disorders include ulcerative colitis and Crohn's disease. Although there is an incomplete understanding of these disorders, they are known to be chronic in nature with episodes of relapse and exacerbation. The exact cause of ulcerative colitis remains unclear; however, hereditary, infectious and immunological factors have been implicated in its profile. The average age group for this disease is approximately 15–35 years.

Crohn's disease is considered to be an autoimmune disease whereby the body's own immune system attacks the GI tract which ultimately causes inflammation. Its classification is a type of inflammatory bowel disease. There has been evidence to suggest a genetic link to the disease, highlighting the risks to individuals and siblings. Males and females are equally affected. The incidence of developing the disease is twofold in people who smoke. Crohn's disease usually presents itself in the teenage years but can occur at any age.

Prednisolone

Prednisolone is a synthetic compound which mimics the actions of corticosteroids. It has an anti-inflammatory and immunosuppressive quality and for this reason is used to treat inflammatory bowel disorders. Dosage may be daily or divided until remission occurs. When this happens prednisolone is withdrawn in reducing doses over a period of days. This drug must not be stopped abruptly without the permission of a doctor as high levels of synthetic steroid ultimately prevent the body from natural steroid production (in essence the body's natural steroid production is switched off in the presence of prednisolone). If prednisolone is abruptly stopped then it may take the brain a number of days to switch the normal level of steroid production on again. As natural steroids are vital for the control of heart rate, blood pressure, salt and water balance,

if these levels are dangerously low then the body can go into crisis which can be rapidly fatal (Addison's crisis).

Mesalazine

Mesalazine is given to relieve symptoms during an acute attack of mainly ulcerative colitis, although it is also used in the treatment of Crohn's disease. In severe cases mesalazine can be given alongside a corticosteroid. It acts directly on inflamed mucosa. This drug can be given as a tablet, suppository or enema. The duration of its action can last for up to 12 hours. Care in administration should be taken with patients suffering renal impairment as the drug has been found to have a correlation with interstitial nephritis (inflammation of the nephrons in the kidney which can lead to kidney failure) with prolonged use.

Case studies

① Mrs Johnson is a 60-year-old widow who has been admitted to the medical assessment unit with a history of stomach pain, nausea and heartburn. She has a past medical history of a gastric ulcer, following the death of her husband five years ago after a terminal illness. Her body mass index (BMI) is >30. She smokes approximately 20 cigarettes a day and describes herself as a bit of a 'stress eater'. After observations of her symptoms she is prescribed a PPI and asked to consider making some lifestyle changes to reduce the reoccurrence of her symptoms. You need to explain to her:

● the action of PPIs on acid secretion;

● the side-effects;

● the lifestyle changes that she should be considering.

② Jack is 18 years old and has been admitted to the medical ward with a history of diarrhoea, weight loss and tiredness. He is diagnosed with Crohn's disease. His father also suffers from this condition. Jack recently started smoking and admits to occasionally binge drinking with his friends. He is finding it very difficult to accept the diagnosis of this long-term condition. The doctor prescribes oral steroid medication and mesalazine (aminosalicylate). You need to explain to Jack:

● what Crohn's disease is;

● the action of steroids and aminosalicylate in regard to Crohn's disease;

● how smoking can affect Crohn's disease.

Key learning points

Introduction

➤ Poor diet and lifestyle are two things that contribute to diseases of the GI tract.
➤ Smoking, alcohol and obesity are the most common risk factors in overproduction of acidity leading to acid reflux of some kind.

Helicobacter pylori

➤ HP is a gram negative microaerophilic (requires oxygen to survive) bacterium that can inhabit various areas of the stomach and duodenum.
➤ Triple therapy eradicates the HP bacteria – antibiotics used alongside a PPI.

Proton pump inhibitors

➤ PPIs include omeprazole, lansoprazole, pantroprazole and rabeprazole. They work by inhibiting gastric acid by blocking the H+/K+ ATP enzyme system (the proton pump) of the gastric parietal cell. They are considered effective, short-term treatments for the use of gastric and duodenal ulcers.

Omeprazole

➤ Omeprazole was the first generic PPI to be introduced, in 2002.

Prostaglandins

➤ Prostaglandins maintain blood flow and protect the stomach lining from the corrosive effects of stomach acid.
➤ COX1 is an enzyme which produces prostaglandins (natural painkillers) in the stomach.
➤ When COX1 is blocked by NSAIDs, inflammation is reduced but the protective mucous lining of the stomach is also reduced which may lead to ulceration and bleeding.

Misoprostol

➤ The action of misoprostol is to reduce the amount of acid that is secreted in the stomach.

Bismuth chelate

➤ Considered cytoprotective, forming a protective barrier over the surface of an ulcer, protecting the gastric mucosa.

Sucralfate

➤ Action is to protect the mucosa from acid-pepsin attack in gastritis and the development of duodenal ulcers.

➢ In an acidic environment it forms a gel with mucous and binds to the ulcer base to form a protective barrier to acid and pepsin.

Irritable bowel syndrome

➢ Characterized by chronic abdominal pain, discomfort, bloating and alteration of bowel habits.

Loperamide

➢ An anti-diarrhoeal drug that reduces the muscular contractions of the intestine and slows down peristalsis.

Codeine phosphate

➢ A weak opioid, producing morphine-like effects and reducing peristalsis.

Mebeverine

➢ Acts directly on the smooth muscle in the gut, causing it to relax. This relieves painful muscle spasms of the gut without affecting its normal motility.

Hyoscine (Baclofen)

➢ Reduces intestinal motility by decreasing the effects of the parasympathetic transmitter acetylcholine on the smooth muscles of the intestines.

Drugs used in inflammatory bowel disorders

➢ Inflammatory bowel disorders include ulcerative colitis and Crohn's disease.
➢ They are known to be chronic in nature with episodes of relapse and exacerbation.

Prednisolone

➢ A synthetic compound which mimics the actions of corticosteroids.
➢ It has an anti-inflammatory and immunosuppressive quality.

Mesalazine

➢ Given to relieve symptoms during an acute attack of mainly ulcerative colitis, although it used in the treatment of Crohn's disease.

Calculations

1 A patient is ordered ranitidine 225mg, orally. The ward is carrying 150mg tablets. How many tablets should be given?

2 A patient requires prednisolone 20mg, once daily. The ward is carrying 5mg tablets. How many tablets should be given?

3 The doctor orders codeine phosphate 30mg four times per day. The ward is carrying 15mg tablets. How many tablets will the patient receive in 24 hours?

4 A patient is prescribed Gaviscon (antacid) 10ml four times per day. How many ml in 24 hours?

5 Mesalazine tablets 400mg have been prescribed six times daily. How many mg is this in 24 hours?

6 A patient is prescribed misoprostal 800mcg daily in four divided doses over 24 hours. Tablet strengths are 200mcg. How often should the tablets be given?

7 A doctor orders hyoscine injection 100mg daily, in divided doses. The ward is carrying 1g/5ml. How many ml in 4g?

8 A patient is prescribed intravenous cimetidine 2.4g daily. The pump should be set to deliver the drug over 24 hours at what dose per hour?

9 Sucralfate suspension is prescribed at 4g daily in divided doses. The ward is carrying 1g/5mL. How many ml in 4g?

10 A doctor prescribes peppermint oil capsules 0.6ml daily in divided doses. The ward is carrying 0.2ml capsules. How many capsules in 24 hours?

For further assistance with calculations, please see Meriel Hutton's book *Essential Calculation Skills for Nurses, Midwives and Healthcare Practitioners* (Open University Press 2009).

Multiple choice questions

1 *Helicobacter pylori*

a) Is a gram negative microaerophilic bacterium
b) Can change its shape from flagella to coccoid
c) Can inhabit the harsh acidic environment of the stomach lining
d) All of the above

2 Peristalsis is controlled by

a) The pituitary gland
b) The hypothalamus
c) The medulla of the brainstem
d) The hippocampus

3 The function of the large intestine is

a) To continue to break down foodstuffs
b) To absorb water and electrolytes from remaining indigestible food
c) To stimulate the pancreas to secrete digestive enzymes
d) To absorb fats

4 The definition of gastritis is

a) Inflammation of the duodenum
b) Inflammation of oesophagus
c) Inflammation of the stomach mucosa
d) Inflammation of the small intestine

5 Chyme is

a) A protein-digesting enzyme.
b) Produced by the parietal cells in the stomach
c) A gastric inhibitory peptide
d) A semi-fluid mass of partially digested food

6 The pH of stomach acid is

a) 1.2–4.0
b) 5.1–7.8
c) 6.2–7.5
d) 4.9–5.2

7 Most absorption takes place in the

a) Stomach
b) Small bowel
c) Liver
d) Gall bladder

8 The taking of food into the mouth is called

a) Digestion
b) Ingestion
c) Absorption
d) Peristalsis

9 What percentage of saliva is made up of water?

a) 60–65%
b) 75–80%
c) 40–55%
d) 90–95%

10 Omeprazole belongs to a group of drugs known as

a) H2 receptor antagonists
b) Proton pump inhibitors
c) Prostaglandins
d) Antacids

Recommended further reading

Anwar, A. (2008) Proton pump inhibitors: use, action and prescribing rationale, *Nurse Prescribing*, 6(1): 26–30.

Barber, P. and Robertson, D. (2012) *Essentials of Pharmacology for Nurses*, 2nd edn. Maidenhead: Open University Press.

Beckwith, S. and Franklin, P. (2007) *Oxford Handbook of Nurse Prescribing*. Oxford: Oxford University Press.

Brenner, G.M. and Stevens, C.W. (2009) *Pharmacology*, 3rd edn. Philadelphia, PA: Saunders Elsevier.

Clayton, B.D. (2009) *Basic Pharmacology for Nurses*, 15th edn. St Louis, MO: Mosby Elsevier.

Coben, D. and Atere-Roberts, E. (2005) *Calculations for Nursing and Healthcare*, 2nd edn. Basingstoke: Palgrave Macmillan.

Downie, G., Mackenzie, J. and Williams, A. (2007) *Pharmacology and Medicines Management for Nurses*, 4th edn. Edinburgh: Churchill Livingstone.

Gatford, J.D. and Phillips, N. (2006) *Nursing Calculations*, 7th edn. Edinburgh: Churchill Livingstone Elsevier.

Greenstein, B. (2009) *Clinical Pharmacology for Nurses*, 18th edn. Edinburgh: Churchill Livingstone.

Greveson, K. (2009) Mesalazine for ulcerative colitis: evidence for use, *Nurse Prescribing*, 7(8): 352–6.

Hutton, M. (2009) *Essential Calculation Skills for Nurses, Midwives and Healthcare Practitioners*. Maidenhead: Open University Press.

Karch, A.M. (2008) *Focus on Nursing Pharmacology*, 4th edn. Philadelphia, PA: Lippincott Williams & Wilkins.

Lapham, R. and Agar, H. (2009) *Drug Calculations for Nurses: A Step-by-step Approach*, 3rd edn. London: Arnold.

Robinson, M. (2005) Proton pump inhibitors: update on their role in acid-related gastrointestinal diseases, *International Journal of Clinical Practice*, 59(6): 709–15.

Simonson, T., Aarbakke, J., Kay, I., Coleman, I., Sinnott, P. and Lyssa, R. (2006) *Illustrated Pharmacology for Nurses*. London: Hodder Arnold.

Starkings, S. and Krause, L. (2010) *Passing Calculation Tests for Nursing Students*. Exeter: Learning Matters.

Drugs used in the treatment of cancer

3

Chapter contents

Learning objectives

After studying this chapter you should be able to:

- Recap the cell cycle.
- Describe symptoms, classification, staging and grading of cancers.
- Outline important issues in the handling of cytotoxic drugs.
- Discuss the general side-effects of cytotoxic drugs.
- Identify the main groups of drugs used as cytotoxic agents.
- Explain the mode of action of akylating, cytotoxic antibiotics, antimetabolites and vinca alkaloids in the treatment of cancer.
- List three categories of drugs that act as antimetabolites.
- Demonstrate an understanding of how tamoxifen and goserelin aid cancer treatment.
- Demonstrate knowledge of the use of steroid drugs in cancer therapy.
- Correctly solve a number of drug calculations with regard to cancer treatment.

41

Introduction

All cancers begin in cells, the body's basic unit of life. To understand cancer, it's helpful to know what happens when normal cells become cancer cells.

The body is made up of many types of cells. These cells grow and divide in a controlled way to produce more cells as they are needed to keep the body healthy. When cells become old or damaged, they die and are replaced with new cells. However, sometimes this orderly process goes wrong. The genetic material *deoxyribonucleic acid* (DNA) of a cell can become damaged or changed, producing mutations that affect normal cell growth and division. When this happens, cells do not die when they should and new cells form when the body does not need them. The extra cells may form a mass of tissue called a tumour.

A tumour can be either benign or malignant. Benign tumours are non-cancerous and are rarely life-threatening. They do not spread (metastasize) to other parts of the body. Many breast lumps, for example, are benign tumours. Malignant tumours are cancerous and can spread to other parts of the body. When a malignant tumour spreads, the malignant cells break off and travel through the blood lymph system to other places in the body to settle and multiply (or metastasize), resulting in a new tumour called a secondary tumour. The name given to the cancer, however, is reflective of its origin, even if it has spread to other areas of the body. For example, if prostate cancer has spread to the liver it is still called metastatic prostate cancer.

In order to understand this process a little more clearly and to appreciate how certain drugs act in the management of malignant disease we must revisit your knowledge of what is known as the cell cycle.

The cell cycle

This is a complex area, so do not be put off. We do not expect you to understand the cell cycle after reading this section once; indeed you may need to read it a number of times before it makes sense to you.

In cells with a nucleus (eukaryotes), the cycle can be divided in two brief periods. The first is called the *interphase*. During this phase the cell grows, accumulating nutrients needed for mitosis (cell division) and duplicating its DNA so there is enough for the new cell. The second period is called *mitosis* or the 'M phase'. During this phase the cell splits itself into two distinct cells, often called 'daughter cells'. The cell division cycle is a vital process by which a single-celled fertilized egg develops into a mature organism, as well as the process by which hair, skin, blood cells and some internal organs are renewed.

Prior to and within interphase and mitosis the cell has what are referred to as 'gaps'. Here they are:

G0 This is the first gap point and is relatively easy to understand. It is the resting phase where the cell has left the cycle and has stopped dividing. The G0 phase occurs prior to the commencement of the interphase.

G1 This is the second gap period and occurs in the interphase. During this gap period, cells increase in size and there is also a control mechanism which comes into play to ensure that everything is ready for DNA production.

S The S stands for *synthesis* and in this phase DNA replication (copying) takes place. This phase also occurs in the interphase period.

G2 This is the last phase to take place in the interphase period. This is the gap between DNA synthesis and mitosis. The cell will continue to grow. There is another cellular control mechanism at this point which ensures that everything is ready to enter the M (mitosis) phase and divide.

M The M stands for mitosis and this is where cell growth stops and cellular energy is focused on the orderly division into two daughter cells. Another control mechanism exists in the mitosis phase which ensures that the cell is ready to complete cell division.

Cells can experience uncontrolled growth if there is damage or mutation to DNA and, therefore, damage to the genes involved in cell division.

Four key types of gene are responsible for the cell division process: *oncogenes* tell cells when to divide; *tumor suppressor genes* tell cells when not to divide; *suicide genes* control apoptosis and tell the cell to kill itself if something goes wrong; and *DNA-repair genes* instruct a cell to repair damaged DNA.

Cancer occurs when a cell's gene mutations make the cell unable to correct DNA damage and unable to commit suicide. Similarly, cancer is a result of mutations that inhibit oncogene and tumor suppressor gene functions, leading to uncontrollable cell growth.

Cancer

There is no single cause for cancer but there are a number of areas that require consideration. Firstly, there is the idea of substances which cause cancer. These are referred to as *carcinogens*. Carcinogens are a group of substances that are thought to be directly responsible for damaging DNA, therefore promoting or aiding cancer. Tobacco, asbestos, arsenic, radiation such as gamma and X-rays, the sun and compounds in car exhaust fumes are all examples of carcinogens. When our bodies are exposed to carcinogens, *free radicals* are formed that attempt to steal electrons from other molecules in the body. These free radicals damage cells and affect their ability to function normally.

Cancer can also be the result of a genetic *predisposition* that is inherited from family members. It is possible to be born with certain genetic mutations or a fault in a gene that makes the person statistically more likely to develop cancer later in life (predisposition). In addition, as we age there is an increase in the number of possible cancer-causing mutations in our DNA. This makes age an important risk factor for cancer.

Finally, several viruses have also been linked to cancer such as human *papillomavirus* (a cause of cervical cancer). In the UK, girls in Year 8 at school (aged 12 to 13) are offered the human papillomavirus vaccine. Girls have three injections over six months given by a nurse. A letter explaining the vaccine and a consent form are sent to the parents before administration of the vaccine. It is up to the individual whether she receives the vaccine.

A two-year 'catch up' programme also began in autumn 2008 to vaccinate girls aged between 13 and 18.

Other important viruses to consider in the initiating of cancer are hepatitis B and C which can cause liver cancer, and Epstein-Barr virus (EBV) (a cause of some childhood cancers). Human immunodeficiency virus (HIV) and anything else that suppresses or weakens the immune system or inhibits the body's ability to fight infections increase the chance of developing cancer.

Symptoms

Cancer symptoms can be quite varied and depend on where the cancer is located, where it has spread to and how big the tumour is. Some cancers are more obvious than others. For example, some can be felt or seen through the skin – a lump on the breast or testicle can be an indicator of cancer in those locations. Skin cancer (melanoma) is often noted by a change in a wart or mole on the skin. Some oral cancers present white patches inside the mouth or white spots on the tongue.

Other cancers have symptoms that are less physically apparent. Brain tumours for example tend to present symptoms early in the disease, but rather than being physically apparent the person may present with symptoms such as a change in cognitive (thinking) or affective (emotional) functions. Pancreatic cancers are often too small to cause symptoms until they cause pain by pushing against nearby nerves or interfere with liver function to cause a yellowing of the skin and eyes called jaundice. Pancreatic tumours may well cause an imbalace in blood sugar levels. This sometimes makes diagnosis difficult.

Symptoms can also result from the growth of a tumour pushing against organs and blood vessels. For example, colon cancers lead to symptoms such as constipation, diarrhoea and changes in stool size. Bladder or prostate cancers cause changes in bladder function such as more frequent (polyuria) or infrequent (oliguria) urination.

As cancer cells use the body's energy and interfere with normal hormone function, it is possible to present symptoms such as fever, fatigue, excessive sweating, anemia and unexplained weight loss. However, these symptoms are common in several other diseases as well. For example, coughing and hoarseness can point to lung or throat cancer as well as several other conditions.

When cancer spreads, or metastasizes, additional symptoms can present themselves in the newly affected area. Swollen or enlarged lymph nodes are common and likely to be present early. There are many lymph nodes all over the body. A cancer cell can be carried to a lymph gland and can become trapped and start another tumour (secondary tumour). Some cancer cells may get into the bloodstream and get carried to other parts of the body where once again they start to grow as a secondary tumour. If cancer spreads to the brain, patients may experience vertigo, headaches or seizures. Spreading to the lungs may cause coughing and shortness of breath. In addition, the liver may become enlarged and cause jaundice, and bones can become painful, brittle and break easily. Symptoms of metastasis ultimately depend on the location to which the cancer has spread.

Cancer classification

Cancers can be grouped under five major headings. These headings come from the type of tissue from which the cancer arises.

- **Carcinomas** are cancers that arise from epitheleal tissue. Epithelial tissue covers the outside of the body and lines organs and cavities. Examples of this type of cancer would be lung, breast and colon cancer.
- **Sarcomas** are cancers that arise from cells that are located in bone, cartilage, fat, connective tissue, muscle and other supportive tissues.
- **Lymphomas** are cancers that begin in the lymph nodes and immune system tissues.
- **Leukaemias** are cancers that begin in the bone marrow and often accumulate in the bloodstream.
- **Adenomas** are cancers that arise in glandular tissue such as in the thyroid, pituitary and adrenal glands.

Cancers are also often referred to by the cell type in which the cancer originated, and carry the suffix -carcinoma or just -oma. For example, haemangio, meaning blood vessel, followed by -oma gives us haemangioma, a cancer arising from blood vessels.

Staging and grading of cancer

The *stage* of a cancer is a measure of how much the cancer has grown and spread. Some cancers are also graded by looking at certain features of the cancer cells using a microscope or other tests. The stage and grade of a cancer help to tell us how 'advanced' it is, and how well it may respond to treatment. As a general guide, the earlier the stage and the lower the grade of a cancer the better the outlook (prognosis).

There are a number of different staging classifications which are used for various cancers. However, one of the simplest and most common is the TNM system. T stands for tumour and refers to how big the tumour has grown. N stands for lymph nodes and indicates if the tumour has spread to the nearest lymph nodes and M stands for metastases – an indication whether the cancer has spread to other parts of the body.

This basic staging goes a step further in that each letter has a number assigned to it indicating the degree of size, involvement and spread. So for example the size of the tumour goes from 0 to 4. A T1 tumour may still exist in the wall of an organ, whereas a T4 tumour would be described as invading nearby structures. Nodes (N) go from 0 to 2. A tumour described as N0 would mean there is no spread to local lymph nodes, whereas an N2 tumour would mean extensive spread. Finally, metastases (M) has a 0–1 scale. An M0 tumour has no metastases present, whereas an M1 tumour means that there is metastasis to some other area of the body such as the brain or liver.

The grading of cancers usually follows a biopsy – a medical test involving the removal of cells or tissues for examination. By examining these cells under a microscope it is possible to grade them as either 'low', 'intermediate' or 'high'. Some cancers may have a slightly different scoring system – for example the Gleason system, which is used to assist in the evaluation of a prognosis for men with prostate cancer. The doctor may well use grading information as well as the stage of the tumour before giving an opinion on the patient's prognosis.

Many management options for cancer exist, including chemotherapy, radiation therapy, surgery, immunotherapy, monoclonal antibody therapy and other methods. Which are used depends on the location and grade of the tumour and the stage of the disease, as well as the general state of a person's health. As this is a pharmacology book, we will now discuss medicines that are used in the management of cancer.

Pharmacological cancer management

The word 'chemotherapy' literally means 'drug treatment' but has almost exclusively become linked to the treatment of cancer. Because the causes of cancer are not always clear and are often complex it is not suprising that the treatment of the disease is complex also, and is overseen by a specialist in this field of medicine. However, you will meet many patients who suffer from cancer – young, old, suffering mental health problems or having a learning disability – and to this end the treatment of cancer is an important aspect of your practice irrespective of which branch of nursing you choose to follow. Therefore some basic understanding of the pharmacology underpinning the treatment of cancer is of the utmost importance to you as a nurse.

Many of the drugs given in the management of cancer are called *cytotoxics*. This name is not used lightly and means 'deadly to cells'. This is important because these drugs have an anti-cancer activity but also destroy *healthy* tissue. Chemotherapy is not always given as a cure, because basically it will not cure all cancers. However, it may be given to prolong a person's life or to help with other effects caused by the tumour (palliative care).

Chemotherapy is often given in combination with other treatments. For example, it can be given prior to radiotherapy or surgery where it may be used to shrink the size of a tumour, therefore giving the other treatments an upper-hand in the destruction of the tumour. It may also be used following treatment by surgery or radiotherapy where the chance of metastasis is high. We have seen a number of patients who have been told that the cancer has been removed only to come back to the hospital a year later with secondary cancers in other parts of their body. If this is to be avoided then chemotherapy is a necessary evil – 'evil' because all drugs used in the chemotherapy of cancer can cause harmful side-effects. As ever, these have to be weighed against the benefit the drugs can have in combating the disease process.

Before we discuss some of the drugs that are used to treat cancer, there are other important issues to bear in mind. The first is the safety of practitioners and patients when preparing and giving cancer medication.

Guidelines for handling cytotoxic drugs

Cytotoxic medication can affect all cells, but tends to affect cells that divide rapidly or uncontrollably, particularly:

- cancerous cells;
- cells from the gastrointestinal (GI) tract;
- hair follicles;
- early blood cells in the bone marrow.

Cytotoxic agents cannot distinguish between normal and malignant cells, although normal cells have a greater capacity for repair. Cytotoxic drugs act by interfering with cell division, but as this action is not specific to tumour cells, normal cells may also be damaged. That is why we discussed the normal cell cycle at the beginning of the chapter. Knowledge of the nature of the cell cycle is necessary to understand the action of cytotoxic medication.

Cytotoxic medication bases its action on the concept of the cell cycle by destroying, damaging or interrupting cellular activity at specific points in the cycle. For health care personnel the potential for exposure exists during tasks such as drug reconstitution, preparation and administration, and disposal of waste equipment or patient waste. Important issues in caring for a person receiving cytotoxic medication are:

- safe handling of cytotoxic medication;
- managing adverse reactions and complications;
- supportive care of the side-effects of cytotoxic drugs.

Direct exposure to cytotoxic drugs can occur during administration or handling, and involves inhalation, ingestion or absorption. The health risk of any procedure involving cytotoxic drugs stems from the inherent toxicity of the drug and the extent to which workers and patients are exposed. Hospitals will require all staff involved with cytotoxic drugs to attend extra training sessions on the handling of these drugs and the management of cytotoxic spillages as part of their orientation and yearly update.

Protective personal equipment such as plastic aprons and gloves is necessary when handling cytotoxic drugs and cytotoxic waste. These measures should be taken by staff handling patient excreta (urine, vomit, faeces) for seven days after the administration of chemotherapy. Families/caregivers should be advised to wear gloves when handling their child's excreta for seven days after the administration of chemotherapy (the use of washing-up gloves or equivalent should be advised in the home). Because cytotoxic therapy can affect the foetus (the drugs are teratogenic – see 'Reproductive function', p. 49), staff who are pregnant or planning to conceive should seek advice from the occupational health department and their line manager before handling any cytotoxic medication.

All cytotoxic spillages should be managed in accordance with national or local policy. In hospitals offering cytotoxic therapy, specialist spillage kits are available and it is up to the nurse to know where these are kept and to use them correctly. Replacement spillage kits are nornally available from the hospital's pharmacy department.

Clinical tip

Above all you must ensure that you have read the policy of the hospital in which you are working for local practices and procedures.

Immediate action in the event of a cytotoxic spillage:

- Restrict access to the spillage area.
- Alert other members of staff in the vicinity and inform a senior member of staff.
- If you have been injured or contaminated, another member of staff must deal with the spillage while you receive attention for the injury or contamination.
- Turn off all fans.
- Obtain and open a cytotoxic spillage kit.
- If protective clothing has been contaminated during the spillage, remove the contaminated items and put on fresh protective clothing from the spillage kit. Place all contaminated items in the 'sharps' bin.

Subsequent action in the event of a cytotoxic spillage:

- Open the cytotoxic spillage kit and follow the procedure as outlined in the pack.
- Any individual who has had any form of contamination from chemotherapy should ensure an incident form is completed and occupational health informed.

- In order to ensure the safety of staff in the event of a subsequent spillage any used kit must be replaced immediately.
- Protective personal equipment must be disposed of in a yellow clinical waste bag. Visors and glasses are often reusable and must be rinsed with warm soapy water.

If there is any cytotoxic residue in or on equipment such as syringes, ampoules, vials or paper waste this must be disposed of in specially designated sharps bins for cytotoxic waste. These bins are usually colour-coded by the hospital so that they are easily recognized.

General side-effects of cytotoxic drugs

Cytotoxic drugs are powerful and often cause unwanted side-effects. We have indicated that these drugs work by killing cells which are dividing and so some normal cells are damaged too. However, side-effects vary from drug to drug. Even with the same drug, different people can react differently. Some people develop more severe side-effects than others who take the same drug. Sometimes, if side-effects are particularly severe, a change to a different drug may be an option.

We will discuss some of the more common side-effects of these drugs before we introduce them individually. Any specific side-effect will be brought to your attention in the relevant section.

Clinical tip

It is important that you inform the patient to ask their doctor or chemotherapy nurse about any side-effects of these drugs as they have the relevant knowledge and experience to give appropriate and evidence-based information and support.

Mouth problems

A painful mouth is a common problem during chemotherapy. A number of drugs can cause this, for example fluorouracil and methotrexate. You will be familiar with methotrexate if you have read

Chapter 5 of *Essentials of Pharmacology for Nurses* (Barber and Robertson 2012). This side-effect is best avoided if possible as once it is established it is more difficult to treat. The key is good oral care both by the patient and by the nurse.

Clinical tip

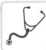

Mouth pain is most effectively avoided by thorough brushing of the teeth. This should be carried out twice a day with a soft toothbrush and fluoride-containing toothpaste. The mouth should rinsed out after meals and at night using water or a 0.9 per cent sodium chloride solution (saline or salt water). Fresh sodium chloride solution for each rinse can be made by dissolving half a teaspoon of salt in 250ml fresh water. The patient can use cool or warm water, whichever they prefer. It is not necessary for them to use antiseptic or anti-inflammatory mouthwashes as there is little evidence that they are any more effective. If the patient has dentures then it is advisable to suggest they continue to clean them as normal.
Pineapple contains an enzyme called ananase. This helps break down protein and milk products and it is therefore helpful to encourage the patient to chew pieces of fresh or unsweetened tinned pineapple. If the patient is taking a drug called fluorouracil, sucking ice cubes during short infusions is a useful measure.

Nausea and vomiting

These side-effects cause a great deal of distress for some individuals. Sometimes the nausea and vomiting may be so distressing that the individual actually refuses any further treatment. Some groups of patients suffer these side-effects more than others, for example, females, those patients above 50 years of age, patients that are anxious and people who tend to suffer from motion sickness. Some patients suffer from more nausea and vomiting as their treatment progresses, and some drugs (e.g. emetogenic drugs) cause more nausea and vomiting than others. For example, flu-orouracil is a mild nausea- and vomit-inducing agent whereas cisplatin is highly emetogenic.

Anti-sickness (antiemetic) medication will usually help and is commonly taken at the same time as, or just before, a cycle of chemotherapy. There are different types of anti-sickness medication. If one does not work well, an alternative may well be available (see Chapter 4).

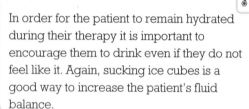

Clinical tip

In order for the patient to remain hydrated during their therapy it is important to encourage them to drink even if they do not feel like it. Again, sucking ice cubes is a good way to increase the patient's fluid balance.

Hair loss (alopecia)

Cytotoxic therapy tends to affect cells that divide rapidly or uncontrollably, particularly hair follicles. Therefore it is hardly surprising that one of its side-effects is to do with the hair itself. Some or all of the patient's hair may fall out. This usually occurs two to three weeks after a course of treatment begins. Body hair and eyelashes may also fall out in addition to scalp hair. After the course of treatment has finished the hair will usually regrow within 4 to 12 months.

Clinical tip

Hair loss bothers some people more than others. The patient may wish to cut their hair short before starting chemotherapy so that any changes are not so dramatic. Some people like to wear a wig. Other people prefer to wear a hat or scarf. In particular, the patient should be reminded to cover their head or wear high protection sunscreen when out in the sun. If their eyelashes fall out, they can wear glasses or sunglasses to protect their eyes on windy days.

Chemotherapy-induced temporary hair loss is one of the most common and distressing side-effects of cancer therapy. If the patient finds the thought of losing their hair very upsetting, the doctor may be able to suggest a treatment that is less likely to cause hair loss. Sometimes there is a choice of drugs that the patient can be prescribed. However, the doctor will want to give the drug that is most likely to work best in treating the patient's cancer. Nevertheless it is always worth the patient discussing this issue with the doctor before commencing therapy.

Hair loss can be reduced by using what is known as a 'cold cap'. This is only suitable for use with certain chemotherapy drugs and certain cancer types. The cold cap lowers the temperature of the scalp which reduces the blood flow. As a result the amount of drug reaching the hair follicles is reduced and the hair is less likely to die off and fall out. However, cold caps do not work for everyone. Clearly, scalp-cooling is undesirable if there is a risk that cancer cells could be present in the blood vessels of the scalp, as these cells are more likely to survive the treatment. The patient cannot wear a cold cap if they are having continuous chemotherapy through a pump because they would have to wear the cap all the time, 24 hours a day.

Unfortunately, even if the patient is able to wear a cold cap it may not work. The patient may still be left with hair thinning and some people still lose their hair completely. You cannot tell whether it will work for you until you try it.

If the patient does elect to have scalp cooling, they will have to spend longer at the hospital having their treatment. They may also have to wear the cold cap for a period before commencing treatment. Cold caps can make the patient feel cold all over and some patients have complained that they cause headaches.

Cold caps are controversial. Some doctors are not happy about their patients using scalp cooling for any type of cancer. The concern relates to the risk of cancer remaining in the scalp; however, there has been very little research into this area and there is not enough evidence to be certain whether scalp cooling is completely safe or not.

Bone marrow suppression

All cytotoxic drugs other than vincristine and bleomycin cause bone marrow suppression. This normally occurs 7 to 10 days after administration of the drug. The bone marrow produces red blood cells, white blood cells and platelets (thrombocytes), therefore the patient may experience problems as a result of depletion in these blood cells.

Firstly, the patient may become anaemic, complain of tiredness and look pale. They may need to have a blood transfusion to correct this problem. There is also an increase in the likelihood of infection due to a drop in white blood cells (leucopenia). Important symptoms here are the development of signs of infection such as fever or a sore throat. The patient may need to receive a high dose of antibiotics directly into their bloodstream if they develop an infection. Finally, bleeding problems can occur. Platelets help the blood to clot and if their number is reduced patients may bruise easily and bleed for longer than usual if they cut themselves. A platelet transfusion may be necessary if the platelet count goes very low.

Prior to each cycle of treatment, it is usual for patients to have a blood test to check their 'blood count'. This establishes the level of their red blood cells, white blood cells and platelets. If any of these is too low, then a treatment cycle may be delayed,

the choice of drugs may be altered or they may be given treatment to boost the levels of these blood constituents.

Reproductive function

Most of the cytotoxic groups of medicines are *teratogenic* which means that they disturb the growth and development of an embryo or foetus. Therefore they should not be administered during pregnancy, especially in the first three months (the first trimester). Advice regarding contraception should also be offered where appropriate before the therapy commences and should continue throughout the treatment and beyond.

Some chemotherapy drugs can affect fertility in both men and women. Sometimes this is temporary and sometimes it is permanent. Treatment regimes that do not contain alkylating agents have a lesser effect on fertility than those that contain this class of drug. If this is a concern, one option may be for men to store sperm or women to store ova (eggs) before chemotherapy treatment begins. These can be 'frozen' and may be able to be used in the future if the patient wishes to have children. Some women develop an early menopause when taking certain cytotoxic drugs.

Extravasation of cytotoxic therapy

Cytotoxic extravasation (tissuing) is the leakage of a cytotoxic drug, which may be given via bolus or infusion, from its intended route into the surrounding tissue. The known incidence of cytotoxic extravasations is relatively low, affecting less than 1 per cent of patients receiving intravenous (IV) cytotoxic chemotherapy, but may be as high as 10 per cent. However, the actual percentage is unknown, since extravasation is often unnoticed and/or undocumented, especially if not severe.

Extravasation of a cytotoxic drug is a serious matter. In particular, the extravasation of vesicant (blister-causing) drugs such as vincristine may lead to widespread tissue necrosis if appropriate action is not taken soon enough. For this reason, it is vital for anyone involved in the IV administration of cytotoxic drugs to have sound theoretical and clinical knowledge of extravasation management. In addition, he or she should be able to identify vesicant and non-vesicant drugs. An excellently and very cleanly placed central line is a huge advantage while infusing vesicant drugs.

Extravasation poses particular dangers. Tissue damage may continue for weeks or even months after such an injury and it can involve nerves and tendons. If appropriate treatment is delayed the patient may need surgical debridement and may even have to have a skin graft. In extreme cases, amputation may be the only option. Any incident of extravasation should be seen as a medical emergency, necessitating a prompt response to minimize damage. Some drugs require other drugs to help with the effects of extravasation – for example, anthracycline extravasation requires prompt administration (within six hours) of a drug called dexrazoxane.

Cytotoxic medication

Generally speaking medicines used in cytotoxic therapy fall into four major groups:

- alkylating drugs;
- cytotoxic antibiotics;
- antimetabolites;
- vinca alkaloids.

Some examples from each of these groups will now be considered

Alkylating drugs

Alkylating agents are one of the earliest and most commonly used chemotherapy agents in the treatment of cancer. They were first introduced in the early 1940s in the form of nitrogen mustards similar to those used in chemical warfare during World War I. Chlorambucil is given orally and is used to treat chronic lymphocytic leukaemia and lymphomas (cancers that begin in the lymphocytes of the immune system and present as a solid tumour of lymphoid cells). This drug causes bone marrow suppression but other side-effects are uncommon.

Cyclophosphamide can be given by mouth or IV infusion. It is also useful in treating lymphomas and leukaemias as well as soft tissue and osteogenic sarcoma (cancer of the bone). One major problem with this drug is that it can cause the bladder to develop a bleeding cystitis. This is rare but can be problematic if cyclophosphamide is given in high doses.

Clinical tip

An increased fluid intake for 24–48 hours after intravenous injection of cyclophosphamide is advised.

Melphalan, procarbazine, thiotepa and busulfan are other examples of alkylating drugs. Although they may differ in their clinical activity, all alkylating agents share the same biochemical mechanism, working directly on the DNA and preventing the cell division process.

Alkylating chemotherapy drugs are effective during all phases of the cell cycle. Therefore they are used to treat a large number of cancers. However, they are more effective in treating slow-growing cancers such as solid tumours and leukaemia. Long-term use of alkylating agents can lead to permanent infertility by decreasing sperm production in males and causing menstruation cessation in females. Many alkylating agents can also lead to secondary cancers such as acute myeloid leukaemia, years after the therapy.

Cytotoxic antibiotics

An early version of cytotoxic antibiotic was the anthracycline group of drugs. Anthracyclines were developed between the 1970s and the 1990s. These compounds are cell-cycle non-specific (i.e. they are effective during all phases of cell cycle) and are used to treat a large number of cancers including lymphomas, leukaemia and uterine, ovarian, lung and breast cancers. Anthracyclines are developed from natural resources. Daunorubicin was discovered by isolating it from soil-dwelling fungus *Streptomyces*. Doxorubicin, which is another commonly used anthracycline chemotherapy agent, is isolated from a mutated strain of *Streptomyces*. Although both of these drugs have similar mechanisms, doxorubicin is more effective in treating solid tumours. Idarubicin, epirubicin and mitoxantrone are other commonly used anthracycline chemotherapy drugs.

Anthracyclines work by forming free radicals (molecules that are very unstable and look to bond with other molecules, destroying their purpose) which break DNA strands thereby inhibiting DNA production and function. Cardiac toxicity is a serious side-effect of anthracyclines as the heart muscle can be damaged.

Cytotoxic antibiotics are widely used to treat and suppress the development of tumours in the body. Similar to anthracyclines, these drugs also form free radicals that break DNA strands, preventing the multiplication of cancer cells. Oncologists usually combine anti-tumour antibiotics with other chemotherapy agents in a treatment regimen.

Bleomycin is one of the most common cytotoxic antibiotics, used to treat testicular cancer and Hodgkin's lymphoma. This drug is usually given either intramuscularly or intravenously. It causes little bone marrow suppression but treatment can result in skin toxicity and pigmentation. Hypersensitivity reactions, such as chills and fever, are also common, particularly a few hours following administration. However, this side-effect can be treated by giving a corticosteroid at the same time as the bleomycin. One particularly difficult side-effect is that bleomycin can lead to *progressive pulmonary fibrosis*. This is an inflammatory lung disorder characterized by abnormal formation of fibrous tissue between the alveoli. Therefore the limiting toxicity for cytotoxic antibiotics tends to be in the lungs; free radicals formed by the cytotoxic antibiotics damage lung cells along with the cancer cells.

Antimetabolites

In order to understand antimetabolites and how they work it is necessary to briefly discuss the processes that are being targeted by these agents. The term 'metabolism' refers to the many chemical reactions that take place in our bodies. We are constantly breaking down food into usable components and using those components to build our proteins, DNA and other cellular structures. 'Metabolite' is a general term for the biological materials that are produced, recycled or broken down in cells. Materials that provide us with key metabolites enter our body as food. These compounds can be broken down into simpler structures that can be reused in our cells. Examples include vitamins and amino acids (the building blocks of proteins). Metabolites that are the end products of a process or pathway may be excreted by the body. An example is urea, the end product of protein metabolism, excreted by the body as a component of urine.

Antimetabolites are structurally similar to metabolites, but they cannot be used by the body in a productive manner. In the cell, antimetabolites are mistaken for the metabolites they resemble, and are processed in a manner similar to normal compounds. The presence of the 'decoy' ('Trojan horse') antimetabolites prevents the cells from carrying out vital functions and the cells are unable to grow and survive. Many of the antimetabolites used in the treatment of cancer interfere with the production of the nucleic acids, ribonucleic acid (RNA) and DNA. If new DNA cannot be made, cells are unable to divide.

There are several different cellular targets for antimetabolites and some common classes of these drugs are folate antagonists, purine antagonists and pyrimidine antagonists.

Folate antagonists

These drugs are also known as 'antifolates'. They work by inhibiting dihydrofolate reductase (DHFR), an enzyme involved in the formation of nucleotides. Nucleotides are molecules that, when joined together, make up the structural units of RNA and DNA. When this enzyme is blocked, nucleotides are not formed, disrupting DNA replication and cell division.

Methotrexate is the primary folate antagonist used as a chemotherapeutic agent and acts at the S phase of the cell cycle. It may be used alone or in combination with other anti-cancer drugs. In 1948, it was found that a diet with reduced levels of folic acid led to a decrease in leukaemia cell counts. That discovery started the search for folate antagonists. The same year, a folate antagonist, aminopterin, was found to produce remissions in childhood leukaemias. Methotrexate was discovered soon after, and proved to be a more effective, less toxic folate analogue. Since then, and despite the isolation of multiple other folate antagonists, methotrexate maintains its significant role as a treatment for breast cancer, osteogenic sarcoma and leukaemias.

This drug is flexible in that it can be given orally, intravenously, intramuscularly or intrathecally (directly into the subarachnoid space). It can cause bone marrow suppression and mucositis, the painful inflammation and ulceration of the mucous membranes lining the digestive tract. However, these side-effects can be lessened by giving the patient folinic acid following the treatment with methotrexate. As this drug is excreted primarily by the kidney its use is contraindicated in those patients who have significant renal/liver impairment. If patients have a pleural effusion (excess fluid that has accumulated in their pleural cavity, the fluid-filled space that surrounds the lungs), or ascites (which is a build-up of excess fluid in the peritoneal cavity), the drug should be avoided. This is because it can accumulate in theses fluids which act as a reservoir for the drug, therefore making the side-effects much more likely.

Purine antagonists

The purines (adenine and guanine) are chemicals used to build the nucleotides of DNA and RNA. The other class of base chemicals, the pyrimidines, are represented in DNA by thymine and cytosine and in RNA by cytosine and uracil (see below).

Before a cell can divide it must duplicate its DNA content, so that each daughter cell has a complete and identical set of genetic information. The duplication process (replication) is like an assembly line, during which nucleotides are joined to each other to form the new DNA molecule.

Phosphate groups and sugar molecules are joined together to create the long strands of DNA found in our chromosomes. The incorporation of a

purine antagonist prevents the continued growth of the DNA and therefore cell division. The purine antagonists function by inhibiting DNA synthesis in two different ways. They can inhibit the production of the purine-containing nucleotides, adenine and guanine. If a cell doesn't have sufficient amounts of purines, DNA synthesis is halted and the cell cannot divide. They may be incorporated into the DNA molecule during DNA synthesis. The presence of the inhibitor is thought to interfere with further cell division.

Mercaptopurine is used as maintenance therapy in patients with acute leukaemias and may also be used in patients suffering with ulcerative colitis or Crohn's disease. Normally a dose of 2.5mg for every kg of body weight is administered. Side-effects include bone marrow suppression.

Fludarabine is used in the initial treatment of advanced B-cell chronic lymphocytic leukaemia. The drug can be given orally or by IV injection or infusion. This drug has a potent and prolonged effect on the bone marrow, making patients more prone to serious infections. Patients may therefore be treated with antibiotics before and during treatment.

Pyrimidine antagonists

The pyrimidine antagonists act to block the synthesis of pyrimidine-containing nucleotides (cytosine and thymine in DNA; cytosine and uracil in RNA). The drugs used to block the construction of these nucleotides have structures that are similar to the natural compound. By acting as 'decoys', these drugs can prevent the production of the finished nucleotides. They may exert their effects at different steps in that pathway and may directly inhibit crucial enzymes. The pyrimidine antagonist may also be incorporated into a growing DNA chain and lead to termination of the process.

For a cell to reproduce, it must first faithfully replicate the entire DNA in its genome. During DNA synthesis, pyrimidine and purine molecules must be made available to allow for the synthesis of the nucleotide building blocks and ultimately the new DNA molecules. A reduction in the availability of the raw materials needed to build DNA, such as that caused by the pyrimidine antagonists, leads to stoppage of DNA synthesis and inhibition of cell division.

As previously noted, cancer cells are often quite rapidly dividing and therefore engaged in DNA synthesis. RNA synthesis is necessary for protein production. The pyrimidine antagonists inhibit the normal processes of DNA and/or RNA synthesis.

Fluorouracil is a drug that has been used for many years in treating cancer. As we have already identified, uracil is a normal component of RNA; therefore the rationale behind the development of this drug was that cancer cells, with their increased genetic instability, might be more sensitive to 'decoy' molecules that mimic the natural compound more than normal cells. The scientific goal in this case was to produce a drug that demonstrated specific uracil antagonism. In the event, fluorouracil proved to have anti-tumour capabilities.

This drug is usually given intravenously and is used to treat a number of solid tumours, such as cancers arising in the GI tract. It may also be used as a cream to treat certain pre-malignant and malignant skin lesions.

A similar drug in this class is capecitabine. Capecitabine is an antimetabolite that is changed to fluorouracil inside the body. It inhibits cell division and interferes with RNA and protein processing. This drug is used to treat metastatic colorectal cancer and metastatic and/or resistant breast cancer and can be given orally. It is often combined with other cytotoxic therapy to achieve the best outcome for the patient.

Vinca alkaloids

The vinca alkaloids are a subset of drugs that are derived from the periwinkle plant, *Catharanthus roseus* (also *Vinca rosea*, *Lochnera rosea* and *Ammocallis rosea*). This plant is also commonly called the Madagascar periwinkle or the rose periwinkle. While it has historically been used to treat numerous diseases, it has most recently been employed for its anti-cancer properties. The plant grows in warm regions of the world and especially in the southern USA. The 'flower' is usually pale pink with a dark violet dot in the centre.

This drug comes from a group called *spindle inhibitors*. Unlike the previous drugs discussed, these agents do not work to alter the DNA structure or function but instead interfere with the mechanics of cell division itself. During mitosis (cell division) the DNA of a cell is replicated and then divided into two new cells. The process of separating the newly replicated chromosomes (the organized structures of DNA and protein that are found in cells) into the two forming cells involves structures called *spindle fibres*. These fibres are constructed with microtubules which attach themselves to the replicated (copied) chromosomes and pull one copy to each side of the dividing cell. Without functional spindle fibres the cell cannot divide and will eventually die. The spindle inhibitor drugs halt division during early mitosis by disabling the movement of chromosomes.

All vinca alkaloids are administered intravenously. They must never be given intrathecally as they are highly neurotoxic and will usually cause death if given in this manner. You may recall the case of Wayne Jowett in 2001 who was supposed to receive a dose of cytosine into spine (intrathecally). However, there was a mistake and vincristine was injected instead and the patient died. Checking of drugs prior to administration is therefore vital and we must make every effort to ensure we do not become complacent.

After injection, vinca alkaloids are eventually metabolized by the liver and excreted. They work in a cell-cycle specific manner and are therefore not active against cells in the resting state.

There are four vinca alkaloids that you may come across in your clinical placements: vinblastine, vincristine, vindesine and vinorelbine. These drugs are used to treat a variety of cancers, including leukaemias, lymphomas, and lung and breast cancers (solid tumours). The patient may complain of peripheral pins and needles (paraesthesia), abdominal pain, constipation and hearing loss (ototoxicity). If the symptoms become severe and the patient displays motor weakness such as a loss of power or difficulty in moving, the therapy may have to be discontinued. Recovery from this assault on the body is slow but is normally complete.

Other drugs used in cancer treatment

Hormonal therapy is one of the major areas of medical treatment for cancer. It involves the manipulation of the endocrine system through the administration of specific hormones, particularly steroid hormones, or drugs which inhibit the production or activity of such hormones (hormone antagonists). Because steroid hormones have a powerful effect on the growth of certain cancer cells, changing the levels or activity of certain hormones can cause certain cancers to cease growing, or even undergo cell death. Surgical removal of endocrine organs, such as orchidectomy (removal of the testes) and oophorectomy (removal of the ovaries) can also be employed as a form of hormonal therapy.

Hormonal therapy is used for several types of cancer that arise from hormonally responsive tissues, including the breast, prostate, endometrium (lining of the uterus) and adrenal cortex. Hormonal therapy may also be used in the treatment of cytotoxic-associated symptoms, such as anorexia. Perhaps the most familiar example of hormonal therapy in oncology is the use of the tamoxifen for the treatment of breast cancer.

Tamoxifen

Tamoxifen is an anti-oestrogen drug that was developed over 30 years ago. It is used widely to treat breast cancer and occasionally some other cancers. Tamoxifen can also be used to treat or prevent the side-effects of breast tenderness and swelling in some men with prostate cancer.

Tamoxifen's action is still not fully understood beyond the fact that as an anti-oestrogen drug it acts against cancers with oestrogen receptors on the surface of their cells (oestrogen-receptor-positive cancers). Tamoxifen fits into the oestrogen receptor but does not activate the cells to divide. The drug stays in place and prevents oestrogen from reaching the cancer cells so that they either grow more slowly or stop growing altogether. Tamoxifen can greatly reduce the chance of oestrogen-receptor-positive cancers coming back after surgery. It can also be used to shrink large tumours before surgery so they can be removed.

This drug is administered orally as a tablet that should be swallowed whole with a glass of water. The tablets come in different strengths: 10, 20 and 40mg. It is also available as sugar-free syrup for people who have difficulty swallowing tablets. Tamoxifen is usually prescribed as a single daily dose and this should be taken at the same time each day. Some women prefer to take the tablet with food as it can cause nausea and leave a metallic taste in the mouth. It is best to advise the patient to find a convenient time of day to take the tablet and stick to it.

Side-effects are more common in pre-menopausal women, who may develop menopausal side-effects as a result of a lowered level of oestrogen. The most common side-effects, apart from nausea are hot flushes and sweats, particularly at night. Sometimes the flushes will gradually lessen over the first few months of treatment but some women continue to have them for as long as they take tamoxifen. There are a number of ways to help reduce or control hot flushes and sweats. Some women find it helpful to avoid or cut down on tea, coffee, nicotine and alcohol. Others seek out complementary remedies (see Chapter 10). There is some evidence that certain antidepressant medicines are proving useful in lessening these symptoms.

Studies have shown that post-menopausal women who take tamoxifen over a long period of time may have a very slightly increased risk of developing cancer of the lining of the womb (endometrial cancer). However, this small risk is generally outweighed by the benefits of taking tamoxifen. As a precautionary measure, in some cancer hospitals women are given regular gynaecological check-ups to detect early signs of endometrial cancer. An ultrasound scan may be performed to check for signs of change in the womb lining. A small probe is inserted into the vagina and the doctor can observe the scan on a screen. Any changes can be seen straight away. This scan is safe and only takes a few minutes.

Aromatase inhibitors

This class of drugs is used in the treatment of breast cancer and ovarian cancer in post-menopausal women. As indicated earlier, breast cancers require quantities of oestrogen in order to grow. In contrast to pre-menopausal women, in whom most of the oestrogen is produced in the ovaries, in post-menopausal women most of the body's oestrogen is produced in the adrenal gland from the conversion of androgens (the chemicals that help produce all oestrogens and the female sex hormones).

The other main source of oestrogen post-menopausally is adipose tissue. Because some breast cancers respond to oestrogen, lowering the oestrogen level in post-menopausal women using aromatase inhibitors has been proven to be effective in breast cancer treatment. Aromatase is an enzyme that produces oestrogen from androgens and adipose tissue. Therefore it would appear reasonable that a drug that inhibits aromatase would have lessening effects on the production of oestrogen in post-menopausal women, and indeed this is the case. Examples of aromatase inhibitors are anastrozole and exemestane.

Gonadorelin analogues

Most prostate cancers need supplies of the male hormone testosterone to grow. Testosterone is produced by the testes and the adrenal glands. The testes will only make testosterone if told to do so by another hormone called the leuteinizing hormone, which is produced in a part of the brain known as the pituitary gland.

Goserelin

Goserelin stops the production of leuteinizing hormone by the pituitary gland. This reduces the production of testosterone. The cancer cells then grow more slowly or stop growing altogether. The cancer may often shrink in size. Goserelin is given by injection under the skin of the abdomen (subcutaneously) every 4 weeks, or as a longer-acting preparation every 12 weeks. The injection is often referred to as an 'implant' and the drug is mixed with oil so that the injections last over a period of time.

Side-effects can occur, and one such is called 'tumour flare'. This means that there may be a temporary increase in the levels of testosterone for the first few days of the treatment. Because of this, the patient may find that they experience an *increase* in symptoms over the first two weeks. They may experience an increase in bone pain or have problems passing urine. Other problems may occasionally occur due to a temporary increase in the size of the tumour. If the patient has any of these problems they should be advised to seek medical help immediately. Other hormonal therapy drugs such as cyproterone acetate, flutamide or bicalutimide may be given for the first few weeks of starting goserelin to prevent tumour flare from occurring.

Loss of sex drive (libido) and erection difficulties (impotence) can occur. These often return to normal after stopping the drug. However, some men may find that these problems continue after the treatment is completed. There may also be an increased risk of developing heart disease or diabetes. However, as in the treatment of breast cancer, the benefits far outweigh the risks involved in taking this medication.

Steroid use in cancer treatment

Steroid preparations help those suffering from cancer in a number of ways. Other than treating cancer, they assist in reducing inflammation, reduce the response of immunity after a transplant, reduce sickness during chemotherapy and help to increase appetite. Steroids contribute to effective treatment of the disease itself by reducing swelling, suppressing allergic reactions, reducing nausea and shrinking the size of a tumour. Examples of steroids used in the treatment of cancer are hydrocortisone, dexamethasone, methylprednisolone and prednisolone. Steroids are injected intravenously or given by infusion, and may also be given in liquid or pill form or as a cream.

Some common side-effects may include indigestion or heartburn, increased appetite, weight gain, swelling at different parts of the body due to water retention, irregular menstruation, mood swings, changes in blood sugar levels, difficulty sleeping and an increased risk of infection.

As is always the case, patients should seek medical advice if they suffer from any of the side-effects, but must *not* discontinue the dose unless recommended to do so. Patients taking steriods must always carry a card whenever they leave home and adopt a strict discipline in adhering to the prescribed regimen (see Chapter 5 of *Essentials of Pharmacology for Nurses*).

Case studies

① A 46-year-old nurse has been diagnosed with breast cancer. She has undergone routine mammography since the age of 40, as her mother and grandmother had breast cancer. The patient has undergone lumpectomy and axillary node dissection. She is currently undergoing cycles of chemotherapy with cyclophosphamide, doxorubicin and fluorouracil. She wants to know the difference between each of the chemotherapeutic drugs being used.

■ What information do you give her?

② Zachary is an active 75-year-old who lives with his wife in a retirement community. He had a heart attack in his fifties, and since then has struggled to lower his high cholesterol and blood pressure. Zachary's wife notices that he gets up frequently during the night to urinate and suggests that he consults a doctor. Zachary agrees to see a urologist and, after a series of tests, is diagnosed with late stage prostate cancer. He is prescribed goserelin, but is unsure what this drug does.

■ Can you explain to him?

Key learning points

Introduction

➢ Cancer occurs when cells do not die when they should and new cells form when the body does not need them. The extra cells may form a mass of tissue called a tumour.

The cell cycle

➢ Four key types of gene are responsible for the cell division process.

Cancer

➢ Carcinogens are a group of substances that are thought to be directly responsible for damaging DNA.

Symptoms

➢ Cancer symptoms can be quite varied and depend on where the cancer is located, where it has spread to, and how big the tumour is.

Cancer classification

➢ Cancers can be grouped under five major headings: carcinomas, sarcomas, lymphomas, leukaemias and adenomas.

Staging and grading of cancer

➢ There are a number of different staging and grading classifications.

Pharmacological cancer management

➢ Many of the drugs given in the management of cancer are called cytotoxics.

Guidelines for handling cytotoxic drugs

➢ Need to safely handle cytotoxic medication.
➢ Need to manage adverse reactions and complications.

General side-effects of cytotoxic drugs

➢ The main side-effects include mouth problems, nausea and vomiting, alopecia, bone marrow suppression and reproductive problems.

Extravasation of cytotoxic therapy

➢ Extravasation means leakage of a cytotoxic drug, which may be given via bolus or infusion, from its intended route into the surrounding tissue.

Cytotoxic medication

➢ There are four major groups: alkylating drugs, cytotoxic antibiotics, antimetabolites and vinca alkaloids.

Alkylating drugs

➢ Commonly used chemotherapy agents which work directly on the DNA and prevent the cell division process.

Cytotoxic antibiotics

➢ Anthracyclines are cell-cycle non-specific (effective during all phases of the cell cycle) and are used to treat a large number of cancers.
➢ Doxorubicin is a commonly used anthracycline chemotherapy agent.

Antimetabolites

➢ Cannot be used by the body in a productive manner.
➢ The presence of the 'decoy' antimetabolites prevents the cells from carrying out vital functions and the cells are unable to grow and survive.

→

←

> Common classes of antimetabolites are: folate antagonists, purine antagonists and pyrimidine antagonists.

Folate antagonists

> Inhibit DHFR, an enzyme involved in the formation of nucleotides.
> Methotrexate is the primary folate antagonist used as a chemotherapeutic agent.

Purine antagonists

> The incorporation of a purine antagonist prevents the continued growth of the DNA and prevents cell division.
> They can inhibit the production of the purine-containing nucleotides, adenine and guanine.

Pyrimidine antagonists

> The pyrimidine antagonists act to block the synthesis of pyrimidine-containing nucleotides.
> By acting as 'decoys', these drugs can prevent the production of the finished nucleotides.

Vinca alkaloids

> These drugs interfere with the mechanics of cell division itself.
> All vinca alkaloids are administered intravenously.

Other drugs used in cancer treatment

> Hormonal therapy is one of the major areas of medical treatment for cancer and is used for several types of cancer that arise from hormonally responsive tissues.

Tamoxifen

> Tamoxifen is an anti-oestrogen drug.
> It is used widely to treat breast cancer.

Aromatase inhibitors

> A class of drug used in the treatment of breast cancer and ovarian cancer in post-menopausal women.
> They work by blocking the enzyme aromatase that produces oestrogen from androgens and adipose tissue.

Gonadorelin analogues

> Goserelin stops the production of leuteinizing hormone by the pituitary gland. This reduces the production of testosterone in men.

→

Steroid use in cancer treatment

➢ Steroids contribute to effective treatment of the disease by reducing swelling, allergic reactions and nausea, and shrinking the size of the tumour.

➢ Some common side-effects include indigestion, increased appetite, weight gain, water retention, irregular menstruation and alteration of mood.

Calculations

1 A patient needs a unit of packed cells over three hours. A unit contains 250ml and the IV set delivers 15 drops/ml. What drip rate in drops per minute is needed?

2 A dose of 750mg vancomycin is to be given. The maximum rate of infusion is 10mg/min. What is the shortest amount of time over which the dose can be given?

3 Your patient is prescribed vancomycin 500mg in 50ml. This dose is to be given over a one-hour period. What would the drops per minute be during this time if the giving set delivers 20 drops per ml?

4 A patient weighs 50kg and has been commenced on busulfan 60mcg per kg. What should be the daily dose in mg based on the patient's weight?

5 Dactinomycin has been prescribed at 15mcg per kg of body weight per day. The child weighs 20kg. What dose of the drug would they receive in a day?

6 A patient has been prescribed doxorubicin intravenously over a four-week treatment cycle. They have been prescribed a dose of 40mg/m^2, the patient's body surface area has been calculated as 1.15m^2. What is the required dose?

7 The paediatric consultant has prescribed vincristine 1.75mg/m^2. The child has a body surface area of 0.40m^2. What dose would be required?

8 Dactinomycin has been prescribed at 400mcg/m^2/per day. The child has a body surface area of 0.825m^2. What dose of the drug would the child receive in a day?

9 A patient has been prescribed panitumumab 75mg to be given intravenously. The dose available on the ward is 0.1g in 5ml. How much will you draw up?

10 A patient is receiving 1L of chemotherapy via a volumetric pump at a rate of 400ml per hour. How long will it take to complete the dose?

For further assistance with calculations, please see Meriel Hutton's book *Essential Calculation Skills for Nurses, Midwives and Healthcare Practitioners* (Open University Press 2009).

Multiple choice questions

1 Which of the following is the correct sequence of the cell cycle?

a) G0, G1, S, G2, M
b) G0, G1, M, G2, S
c) G1, S, G2, M, G0
d) G1, G2, S, M, G0

2 The TNM cancer classification means

a) Tumour, necrosis, mass
b) Tumour, non-invasive, movement
c) Tumour, lymph nodes, metastases
d) Tumour, number, malignancy

3 What type of tissue do adenomas arise from?

a) Muscular
b) Nervous
c) Epithelial
d) Glandular

4 Alkylating drugs stop cell division by their affects on

a) RNA
b) DNA
c) ATP
d) ADP

5 Anthracyclines belong to which group of chemotherapeutic drugs?

a) Alkylating agents
b) Pyrimidine antagonists
c) Cytotoxic antibiotics
d) Vinca alkaloids

6 Fluorouracil is an example of a

a) Pyrimidine antagonist
b) Purine antagonist
c) Folate antagonist
d) Cytotoxic antibiotic

→

7 Vinca alkaloids are derived from which plant?

a) Willow
b) Clover
c) Foxglove
d) Periwinkle

8 Gonadorelin analogues are used in the treatment of which cancer?

a) Liver
b) Bowel
c) Prostate
d) Breast

9 Which of the following drugs is an example of hormone therapy?

a) Methotrexate
b) Capecitabine
c) Vincristine
d) Tamoxifen

10 Which of the following would be described as an antimetabolite?

a) Gonadorelin analogue
b) Aromatase inhibitors
c) Purine antagonist
d) Steroids

Recommended further reading

Barber, P. and Robertson, D. (2012) *Essentials of Pharmacology for Nurses*, 2nd edn. Maidenhead: Open University Press.

Beckwith, S. and Franklin, P. (2007) *Oxford Handbook of Nurse Prescribing*. Oxford: Oxford University Press.

Brenner, G.M. and Stevens, C.W. (2009) *Pharmacology*, 3rd edn. Philadelphia, PA: Saunders Elsevier.

Clayton, B.D. (2009) *Basic Pharmacology for Nurses*, 15th edn. St Louis, MO: Mosby Elsevier.

Coben, D. and Atere-Roberts, E. (2005) *Calculations for Nursing and Healthcare*, 2nd edn. Basingstoke: Palgrave Macmillan.

Dougherty, L. (2008) IV therapy: recognizing the differences between infiltration and extravasation, *British Journal of Nursing*, 17(14): 896.

Downie, G., Mackenzie, J. and Williams, A. (2007) *Pharmacology and Medicines Management for Nurses*, 4th edn. Edinburgh: Churchill Livingstone.

Gatford, J.D. and Phillips, N. (2006) *Nursing Calculations*, 7th edn. Edinburgh: Churchill Livingstone Elsevier.

Greenstein, B. (2009) *Clinical Pharmacology for Nurses*, 18th edn. Edinburgh: Churchill Livingstone.

Hutton, M. (2009) *Essential Calculation Skills for Nurses, Midwives and Healthcare Practitioners*. Maidenhead: Open University Press.

Ismael, G., Rosa, D., Mano, M. and Awada, A. (2008) Novel cytotoxic drugs: old challenges, new solutions, *Cancer Treatment Reviews*, 34(1): 81–91.

Karch, A.M. (2008) *Focus on Nursing Pharmacology*, 4th edn. Philadelphia, PA: Lippincott Williams & Wilkins.

Lapham, R. and Agar, H. (2009) *Drug Calculations for Nurses: A Step-by-step Approach*, 3rd edn. London: Arnold.

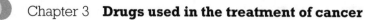

Lomas, C. (2008) Tamoxifen management needed, *Nursing Times*, 104(45): 6.

Lomas, C. (2008) Chemotherapy risks understated, *Nursing Times*, 104(46): 7.

Pattison, J. (2002) Managing cytotoxic extravasation, *Nursing Times*, 98(44): 32–4.

Silvis, N. (2001) Antimetabolites and cytotoxic drugs, *Dermatologic Clinics*, 19(1): 105.

Simonson, T., Aarbakke, J., Kay, I., Coleman, I., Sinnott, P. and Lyssa, R. (2006) *Illustrated Pharmacology for Nurses*. London: Hodder Arnold.

Starkings, S. and Krause, L. (2010) *Passing Calculation Tests for Nursing Students*. Exeter: Learning Matters.

Drugs used in the treatment of nausea and vomiting

4

Chapter contents

Learning objectives

After studying this chapter you should be able to:

- Describe the vomiting reflex.
- Explain the neuronal pathways, transmitters and receptors involved in nausea and vomiting.
- List the causes of nausea and vomiting.
- Demonstrate an overview of the drug treatment of nausea and vomiting.
- Discuss drugs that are used to treat nausea and vomiting in pregnancy.
- Describe drugs that are used to treat post-operative nausea and vomiting.
- Define what is meant by viral disease.
- Demonstrate an understanding of the drugs used to treat nausea and vomiting in cytotoxic chemotherapy.
- Identify the main drugs used to treat motion sickness.
- Explain simply how the inner ear functions.
- Demonstrate an understanding of the antiemetics used in the management of Ménière's disease.
- Correctly solve a number of drug calculations with regard to antiemetics.

Introduction

Nausea and vomiting are biological defence mechanisms. The major physiological function of emesis (vomiting) is to remove toxic or harmful substances from the body after ingestion. However, emesis is multifactorial in origin and can be caused by a range of stimuli, including medical interventions, some of which apparently have little to do with ingesting poisonous substances. In addition to poison ingestion and gastroenteritis, emetic stimuli include motion, surgery, pregnancy, various drugs and radiation. Disgusting sights, smells or memories can also cause nausea and vomiting, and this has a physiological basis leading to avoidance.

Nausea and vomiting are distressing to patients but they can also be a problem clinically. For example, post-operative nausea and vomiting is common and can result in extended hospital stays, increased bleeding, aspiration pneumonia and even the reopening of surgical wounds as a result of the involuntary muscular contractions associated with vomiting. Nausea and vomiting constitute one of the most severe side-effects of cancer chemotherapy (see Chapter 3). The fear of chemotherapy-induced nausea and vomiting can result in patients receiving sub-optimal doses of chemotherapy and the conditioned response of anticipatory nausea and vomiting can even result in up to 25 per cent of patients refusing chemotherapy treatment. Nausea and vomiting also impose an economic burden on the health care system as a result of the time spent cleaning up, potential delays in recovery and discharge, and increased medical care.

The vomiting reflex

The process of emesis can be classified into three phases: nausea, retching and vomiting. Nausea is described as an unpleasant sensation that immediately precedes vomiting. A cold sweat, pallor, salivation, a noticeable disinterest in the surroundings, loss of gastric tone, duodenal (first portion of the small intestine) contractions and the reflux (movement) of intestinal contents into the stomach often accompany nausea.

Retching follows nausea, and comprises laboured spasmodic respiratory movements against a closed glottis with contractions of the abdominal muscles, chest wall and diaphragm without any expulsion of gastric contents. Retching can occur without vomiting but normally it generates the pressure that leads to vomiting.

Vomiting is caused by the powerful sustained contraction of the abdominal and chest wall musculature, which is accompanied by the descent of the diaphragm and the opening of the gastric cardiac sphincter. The cardiac sphincter is a band of muscle that normally stops gastric content from entering the oesophagus during digestion. This is a reflex activity that is not under voluntary control. It results in the rapid and forceful evacuation of stomach contents up to and out of the mouth. Figure 4.1 shows the act of vomiting in more detail.

Receptors that respond to movement (mechanoreceptors) and receptors that respond to chemicals (chemoreceptors) located in the stomach, jejunum (second portion of the small intestine) and ileum (third portion of the small intestine) are involved with the detection of emetic stimuli in the gastrointestinal (GI) tract. Mechanoreceptors are tension receptors that initiate emesis in response to distension and contraction (e.g. from bowel obstruction). Chemoreceptors respond to a variety of toxins in the intestinal lumina. It is thought that the afferent (ingoing) neuronal pathways from the abdomen are the same regardless of the stimulus.

The final common pathway for efferent (outgoing) responses that produce emesis is the vomiting centre which controls the act of vomiting. Numerous neuronal pathways converge on the vomiting centre in the medulla (part of the hind brain) where the vomiting reflex is initiated. The vomiting centre is not a discrete anatomical site, but represents interrelated neuronal networks. Inputs to the vomiting centre include vagal sensory pathways from the GI tract. This means that the vagus nerve carries certain sensations from the GI tract to the vomiting centre and excites it. Neuronal pathways from the labyrinths, higher centres of the cortex, intracranial pressure receptors and the chemotactic trigger zone all play a role in exciting the vomiting

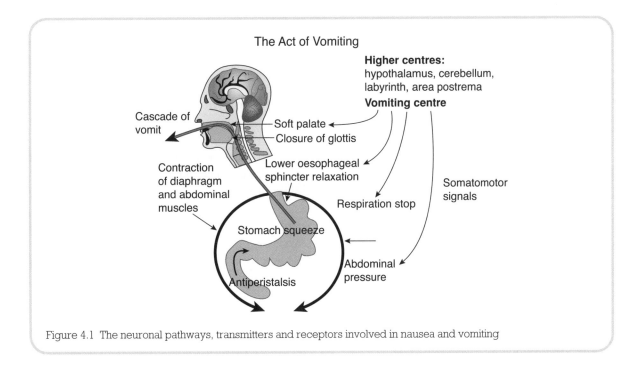

The Act of Vomiting

Higher centres:
hypothalamus, cerebellum,
labyrinth, area postrema
Vomiting centre

Cascade of vomit

Soft palate
Closure of glottis

Contraction of diaphragm and abdominal muscles

Lower oesophageal sphincter relaxation

Somatomotor signals

Respiration stop

Stomach squeeze

Abdominal pressure

Antiperistalsis

Figure 4.1 The neuronal pathways, transmitters and receptors involved in nausea and vomiting

centre. When activated, the vomiting centre induces vomiting via stimulation of the salivary and respiratory centres and the pharyngeal, GI and abdominal muscles.

The chemotactic trigger zone (CTZ) acts as the entry point for emetic stimuli and humoral substances (emetic chemicals carried in the blood). The CTZ is outside the blood-brain barrier (BBB) and therefore responds to stimuli from either the cerebral spinal fluid (CSF) or the blood.

A wide variety of receptor types and neurotransmitters are found in areas of the brain thought to control vomiting, and each may have a role in emesis. Peripheral receptors in the GI tract are also involved. The neurotransmitters include histamine, acetylcholine, dopamine, noradrenaline, adrenaline, 5-hydroxytryptamine (5-HT or serotonin) and substance P (found in chronic pain pathways). In support of their role in emesis, it has been shown that drugs which block the receptors for each of these transmitters have antiemetic effects.

The main classes of antiemetic drugs commonly used are shown in Box 4.1, although it should be appreciated that many drugs have multiple mechanisms of action.

Box 4.1 Main classes of antiemetic drugs

Class	Drug
Anticholinergics	Scopolamine (L-hyoscine)
Antihistamines	Cinnarizine Cyclizine Promethazine
Dopamine antagonists	Metoclopramide Domperidone Droperidol (withdrawn 2001) Haloperidol
Cannabinoids	Nabilone
Corticosteroids	Dexamethasone
Histamine analogues	Betahistine
5-HT$_3$-receptor antagonists	Granisetron Ondansetron Tropisetron

The causes of nausea and vomiting

A wide range of pathological and physiological conditions can induce nausea and vomiting. The most prevalent of these are summarized in Box 4.2.

Box 4.2 Major causes of nausea and vomiting

Drug/ treatment-induced	Cancer chemotherapy
	Opiates
	Nicotine
	Antibiotics
	Radiotherapy
Labyrinth disorders	Motion
	Ménière's disease
Endocrine causes	Pregnancy
Infectious causes	Gastroenteritis
	Viral labyrinthitis
Increased intracranial pressure	Haemorrhage
	Meningitis
Post-operative	Anaesthetics
	Analgesics
	Procedural
Central nervous system causes	Anticipatory
	Migraine
	Bulimia nervosa

Management of nausea and vomiting

There are three very important underlying principles when it comes to managing nausea and vomiting in patients.

- Identification and elimination of the underlying cause if possible.
- Control of the symptoms if it is not possible to eliminate the underlying cause.
- Correction of electrolyte, fluid or nutritional deficiencies.

It is important to care for the well-being and comfort of the patient, since poor management of this can lead to delayed recovery, poor clinical outcome and refusal of future treatment.

Drug treatment

The drug treatment of nausea and vomiting is shown in Figure 4.2. A wide range of drugs has been shown to have effects on nausea and vomiting. These include antihistamines, anticholinergics (which block the effects of acetylcholine), dopamine receptor antagonists, 5-HT$_3$ receptor (serotonin) antagonists, cannabinoids, benzodiazepines, corticosteroids and gastroprokinetic agents (which enhance the movement of the small intestine). Each drug affects different receptors, and some act at a number of different sites. This determines their different clinical uses. For example, the 5-HT$_3$ antagonists are effective in chemotherapy- and radiation-induced nausea and vomiting but do not inhibit nausea and vomiting resulting from the use of opiates or motion. On the other hand, antihistamines provide effective control of post-operative nausea and vomiting, and emesis resulting from opioids or motion but are less effective against nausea and vomiting from aggressive cancer chemotherapy

A multi-drug approach to the treatment of different types of nausea and vomiting is often used in clinical practice, based on knowledge of the causes of the underlying nausea and vomiting and the sites of action of each of the available drugs (see Figure 4.2).

Nausea and vomiting in pregnancy

Nausea and vomiting in pregnancy is a common occurrence, as we are sure all mothers will testify to. However, the severity of these symptoms can vary. 'Morning sickness' describes mild nausea and vomiting which often develop by the time the individual is 5 to 6 weeks pregnant. The symptoms are generally worse around 9 weeks, and typically improved by 16 to 18 weeks. However, symptoms can continue until the third trimester (six to nine months) in 15 to 20 per cent of women and until

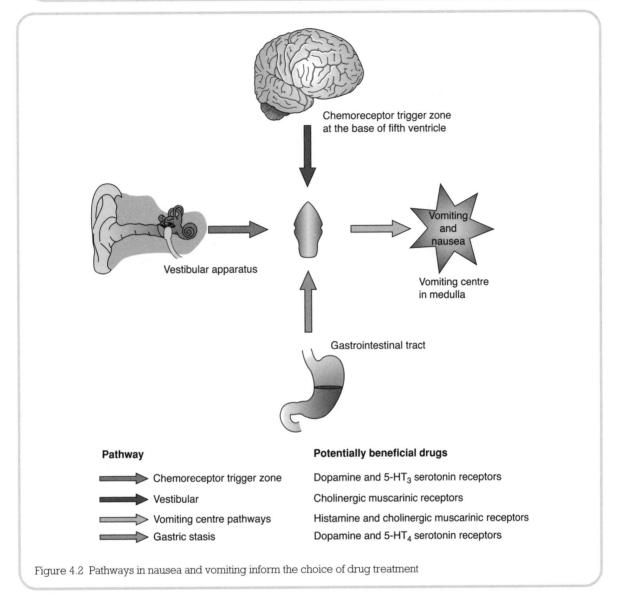

Figure 4.2 Pathways in nausea and vomiting inform the choice of drug treatment

delivery in 5 per cent. Despite the name, a woman may feel sick at any time of day and many women (80 per cent) feel sick throughout the day. It is interesting to note that women who suffer mild nausea and vomiting during their pregnancy have fewer miscarriages and stillbirths than women without these symptoms (Harker et al. 2004).

A less well-known term is 'hyperemesis gravidarum', which is used to describe a more severe condition where the woman may be vomiting many times during the day and losing weight. This condition usually requires the person to be admitted to hospital. Women with hyperemesis often vomit every day and may lose more than 5 per cent of their pre-pregnancy body weight. In most cases, women with this condition will have blood and urine tests that show evidence of dehydration.

The cause of pregnancy-related nausea and vomiting is not clear. Several theories have been proposed although none have been definitively proven. Increased hormone levels, slowed movement of the stomach contents and psychological factors are among the more common theories.

However, the woman is more likely to develop nausea and vomiting during pregnancy if:

- she has suffered it during a previous pregnancy;
- she suffers from sickness while taking oestrogen (e.g. contraceptive pills);
- she suffers from motion sickness (travel sickness).

The aim in treating nausea and vomiting in pregnancy is to help the woman feel better and to allow her to eat and drink so that she does not become dehydrated or start to lose weight. Before considering the use of medication, advice regarding dietary changes should be given. One of the most important things to remember is to avoid anything that will trigger the person's nausea and vomiting. Triggers can be odours, stuffy rooms, noise or simply being tired.

Clinical tip

Encourage the partient to try to eat before or as soon as they feel hungry to avoid an empty stomach, which may aggravate nausea. Eating snacks frequently and having small meals that are high in protein or carbohydrates and low in fat may be of benefit. When drinking it is helpful to advise the patient to drink cold, clear and carbonated or sour fluids (e.g. ginger ale, lemonade), and to take these in small amounts between meals. Smelling fresh lemon, mint or orange, or using an oil diffuser with these scents, may also be helpful in reducing nausea. Eliminating spicy foods helps some women as does brushing the teeth following eating and avoiding changing position quickly.

Most pregnant women manage to eat and drink enough and therefore do not need the intervention of antiemetic drugs. However, these drugs are advisable if symptoms are persistent and severe and do not minimize when the above responses have been adopted.

It is generally best to avoid giving medicines to pregnant women, and the example of thalidomide is a cautionary one. This drug was used as an antiemetic in the 1950s and sold in a number of countries across the world from 1957 until 1961 when it was withdrawn from the market after being found to be a cause of birth defects. However, some drugs have been used for a number of years to treat nausea and vomiting due to pregnancy and are believed to be safe.

Promethazine

This drug is used to combat moderate to severe morning sickness and hyperemesis gravidarum. In the UK promethazine is the drug of first choice, being preferred as an older drug with which there is a greater experience of use in pregnancy (second-line choices being metoclopramide or prochlorperazine).

Promethazine is a phenothiazine in the same drug class as chlorpromazine and trifluoperazine (see Chapter 8 of *Essentials of Pharmacology for Nurses*). However, unlike the other drugs in this class, promethazine is not used as an antipsychotic. It is used as an antihistamine, a sedative and an antiemetic. The body releases histamine during several types of allergic reaction. When histamine binds to its receptors on cells it stimulates changes within the cells that lead to sneezing, itching and increased mucous production. Antihistamines such as promethazine compete with histamine for one of the receptors for histamine (the H_1 receptor) on cells. When the antihistamines bind to the receptors they do not stimulate the cells but do prevent histamine from binding with and stimulating the cells. Promethazine also blocks the action of acetylcholine (the 'anticholinergic effect') and this may explain its benefit in reducing nausea in pregnancy. It also has a sedative action.

The drug comes in tablets, and can also be administered intramuscularly and as suppositories. The dose normally starts at 25mg and is administered at bedtime. The dose may be increased at a doctor's discretion.

Clinical tip

The bedtime dosing of promethazine is important because sedation is often a side-effect.

Prochlorperazine

Similar to promethazine, prochlorperazine has two quite different uses. In higher doses it is used in the treatment of psychiatric illnesses. In lower doses it is used in the management of nausea and vomiting. Prochlorperazine works by blocking dopamine receptors in the brain. Dopamine is a natural compound called a neurotransmitter and is involved in transmitting messages between brain cells. Dopamine is known to be involved in regulating mood and behaviour, among other things.

Prochlorperazine controls nausea and vomiting by blocking dopamine receptors found in the CTZ. This prevents the CTZ from sending messages to the vomiting centre that would otherwise cause nausea and vomiting. This drug should only be used under the supervision of a doctor and can be excreted in breast milk.

Metoclopramide

Metoclopramide is called a 'prokinetic' drug because it stimulates the muscles of the GI tract, including the muscles of the lower oesophageal sphincter, stomach and small intestine, by interacting with receptors for acetylcholine and dopamine on GI muscles and nerves.

The lower oesophageal sphincter, located between the oesophagus and the stomach, normally prevents reflux of acid and other contents in the stomach from backing up into the oesophagus. In patients with gastro-oesophageal reflux disease (GORD), a weakened lower oesophageal sphincter allows reflux of stomach acid into the oesophagus, causing heartburn and damage to the oesophagus (oesophagitis). Metoclopramide decreases the reflux of stomach acid by strengthening the muscle of the lower oesophageal sphincter. Metoclopramide also stimulates the muscles of the stomach and thereby hastens emptying of solid and liquid meals from the stomach into the intestines.

This medicine comes as tablets and syrup and can also be administered via intramuscular (IM) injection. It has long been used in all stages of pregnancy with no evidence of harm to the mother or unborn baby. However, as with both the other drugs discussed in this section, it does cross into breast milk. Metoclopramide is generally well-tolerated when used in low doses for brief periods. Neurological side-effects increase with higher doses and longer periods of treatment.

Clinical tip

When used in pregnancy metoclopramide is monitored carefully and only the the lowest dose to control symptoms is used. It may impair the mental and/or physical abilities to drive or operate machinery. Therefore it is best administered before sleep.

Post-operative nausea and vomiting

There is no clear indication as to the chances of a person becoming nauseated or vomiting following surgery. Post-operative nausea and vomiting is described as being distressing by patients at a time when they are already feeling very uncomfortable, anxious and vulnerable. They quite naturally are going to feel embarrassed by vomiting in the presence of staff and other patients, and by the need for hospital staff to clear up after them. Previous experience of post-operative nausea and vomiting can make an individual anxious at the thought of going through the same thing again, and indeed anticipatory nausea and vomiting may add to the risk of further occurrences. Post-operative nausea and vomiting can have such a profound effect on some patients that they are reported to be more willing to suffer a degree of pain in preference to experiencing it.

Not only is post-operative nausea and vomiting detrimental to the patient psychologically, it also has serious physical consequences. The powerful muscular contractions present when someone vomits can lead to damage of wound stitching, so causing the risk of bleeding. A further complication comes from the increased risk that the patient may inhale the gastric contents into the lungs, leading to respiratory obstruction, pulmonary inflammation or, worse still, aspiration pneumonia. Severe vomiting can lead to electrolyte imbalance or simply affect the patient's appetite. Both these are problem areas when recovering from surgery.

There is also a cost to the NHS. This problem has been highlighted as the most common reason for patients having to stay in hospital longer than planned, making its management of great importance to the patient and to the hospital budget.

Deciding which antiemetic to use can be troublesome because the exact involvement of each neuronal pathway, transmitter and receptor in nausea and vomiting is not known and it is likely to vary with the surgical procedure and drugs employed. Activation of the CTZ by anaesthetics, opioids and humeral factors released during surgery is thought to be important, as is activation of the labyrinths and GI tract resulting from surgical manipulation.

Because no currently available antiemetic is especially effective by itself, and successful control is often elusive, a multimodal approach is frequently taken. Promethazine, prochlorperazine and metoclopramide can all be used in post-operative nausea. Other suitable drugs include the following.

Ondansetron

Chemotherapy, radiotherapy and surgery can cause a substance called serotonin (5-hydroxytryptamine or 5-HT) to be released in the gut. In turn 5-HT acts on the 5-HT$_3$ receptors that are found in the gut and causes nerve messages to be sent to the vomiting centre. Serotonin released by chemotherapy, radiotherapy and surgery also activates the 5-HT$_3$ receptors that are found in the CTZ, causing further messages to be sent to the vomiting centre.

Ondansetron works by blocking the 5-HT$_3$ receptors that are found in the brain and gut. This prevents the nausea messages being sent from these areas to the vomiting centre. Ondansetron therefore prevents nausea, retching and vomiting that can otherwise occur following surgery or due to cancer treatment.

Ondansetron can be administered by mouth as tablets or syrup, by IM injection, by intravenous (IV) infusion or by suppository. This drug is generally not administered to patients who have an allergy to other 5-HT$_3$ antagonists (e.g. granisetron), those with a decreased liver function, blockage of the gut (intestinal obstruction) or disturbance of salt levels (electrolytes) such as potassium, sodium and magnesium in the blood, those with a history of heart problems and those with irregular heartbeats (arrhythmias). It should also be avoided by people taking drugs to treat arrhythmia or beta-blocker medicines.

Cyclizine

Cyclizine lactate can be used before emergency surgical procedures to help prevent vomiting and aspiration of gastric contents. It may be given after surgery to relieve nausea and vomiting caused by general anaesthetics or strong painkillers such as opioids administered during surgery. Cyclizine is an antihistamine which directly affects CTZ and in this way blocks histamine from triggering the vomiting reflex. It works in the same way as promethazine.

Cyclizine may be given orally as 50mg tablets three times daily. If the patient is nauseous and vomiting it may be given as an IM or IV injection of 50mg up to three times daily. In children of 6–12 years the dose is halved to 25mg three times daily.

Cyclizine has effects on a number of body systems. Its action on the nervous system may produce drowsiness and sedation in many patients. Motor skills may be impaired and, conflictingly, in some patients the drug may cause restlessness, excitation, nervousness and insomnia. However, this is very rare in comparison to the sedative effects. Cardiovascular side-effects have included hypotension, tachycardia and palpitations. Cardiovascular changes recorded after IV administration have included an increase in heart rate, a decrease in cardiac output and a decrease in blood pressure, although this is rare. GI side-effects are mild in nature and include nausea, dry mouth and constipation.

Ocular side-effects can involve blurred vision, double vision (diplopia) and dry eyes due to the anticholinergic effects of the drug. Therefore it should not be given to patients with closed angle glaucoma. Glaucoma is a disease in which the optic nerve is damaged, leading to progressive, irreversible loss of vision. It is often, but not always, associated with increased pressure of the fluid in the eye. The anticholinergic effects of cyclizine tend to raise the occular pressure. In addition these anticholinergic effects can have genitourinary side-effects such as urinary retention. The drug is therefore not given to patients who have prostatic enlargement (hypertrophy).

Nausea and vomiting in cytotoxic chemotherapy

Cytotoxic chemotherapy is renowned for nausea and vomiting as side-effects. The acute phase of emesis in chemotherapy responds well to 5-HT$_3$ antagonists like ondansetron; however, emesis in cytotoxic chemotherapy has what is known as a delayed phase (vomiting two to five days following commencement of treatment) and this remains difficult to control. The discovery and development of neurokinin (NK$_1$) receptor antagonists has elicited antiemetic effects in both the acute and especially in the delayed phases of emesis.

This group of drugs blocks the actions at neurokinin receptors in both the CTZ and the vomiting centre. The drug is given along with a 5HT$_3$ antagonist such as ondansetron and a corticosteroid in the treatment of nausea and vomiting induced by cisplatin.

Aprepitant

Aprepitant comes as a capsule to take by mouth. To prevent nausea and vomiting caused by cancer chemotherapy, it is usually taken once daily, with or without food, during the first few days of the treatment.

> **Clinical tip**
>
> Aprepitant is usually given one hour before the first dose of chemotherapy, and then each morning for the next two days.

Aprepitant capsules come in two different strengths. The doctor may prescribe both, for the patient to take at different times. The patient must be advised to take the right strength at the right time as directed.

Aprepitant is usually used only during the first three days of the treatment cycle. An IV formulation of this drug is known as fosaprepitant, which is converted into aprepitant once it is in the body. This drug is administered over 15 minutes, starting about 30 minutes before chemotherapy, together with a serotonin (5-HT$_3$) receptor antagonist and a steroid such as dexamethasone.

> **Clinical tip**
>
> It is important not to take this medicine when receiving other drugs. Aprepitant/fosaprepitant should not be prescribed if the patient is taking pimozide.

Aprepitant may raise pimozide in the blood to dangerous levels. It is also important to advise women taking the oral contraceptive that aprepitant may cause the birth control pills not to work. Backup methods of birth control should be used during treatment and for one month after the last dose of this drug.

The drug has an effect on the levels of warfarin in those individuals taking this drug, causing them to lower. Therefore if the patient is taking warfarin they will need their International Normalized Ratio (INR) checking frequently. The patient should also make sure the doctor knows that they are taking both types of tablet.

As with most drugs, side-effects do occur and these range from fatigue and listlessness, constipation, loss of appetite and pain at the injection site to more serious effects such as allergic reactions.

Motion sickness

Motion sickness is also known as *kinetosis*, and most of us have heard it called 'travel sickness'. It is a condition in which a disagreement exists between visually perceived movement and the vestibular system's sense of movement. Depending on the cause it can also be referred to as 'seasickness', 'car sickness', 'simulation sickness', 'airsickness' and even 'spacesickness'. Many people are susceptible to motion sickness even in mild circumstances such as being on a boat in calm water, although the symptoms will greatly increase in more severe conditions.

The most common symptoms of motion sickness are dizziness, tiredness and nausea. There is also a collection of symptoms called *sopite syndrome* in which a person feels fatigue or tiredness in association with motion sickness. If the motion causing nausea is not resolved, the sufferer will frequently vomit. Unlike ordinary sickness, vomiting in motion sickness tends not to relieve the nausea.

The most common theory for the cause of motion sickness is that it functions as a defence mechanism against toxins that may be released to attack the nervous system (neurotoxins). The CTZ is responsible for inducing vomiting when poisons are detected, and for resolving conflicts between vision and balance. When feeling motion but not seeing it (e.g. in a ship with no windows), the inner ear transmits to the brain that it senses motion, but the eyes tell the brain that everything is still. As a result of this argument, the brain will come to the conclusion that one of our senses must be making it up (hallucinating) and further conclude that the hallucination is due to poison ingestion. The brain therefore responds by inducing vomiting to clear the supposed toxin. In the case of car sickness, a visual stimulus moving by outside the vehicle creates visual sensory conflict, because the rest of the body senses it is still.

One of the most effective drugs used in the treatment of motion sickness is hyoscine.

Hyoscine

Hyoscine is one of the best medicines for preventing travel sickness and is derived from plants. It works by blocking the confusing nerve signals from the patient's vestibular system. Hyoscine tablets are available over the counter at a pharmacy and should be taken about 30 minutes before travel. They last for four to six hours. The dose for an adult by mouth would be 300mcg before the journey followed by 300mcg six-hourly if required. A maximum of three doses should be taken in a 24-hour period. For a child of 4–10 years a dose of 75–150mcg is appropriate, and in children over 10 this can be increased to 150–300mcg.

Hyoscine can also be prescribed by a doctor as a skin patch. The patient sticks it onto the skin behind their ear five or six hours before travelling, and the patch can prevent travel sickness for up to 72 hours. However, patches are only suitable for adults and children over the age of 10. Hyoscine may cause side-effects such as drowsiness, blurred vision and dizziness, therefore patients should not drive or operate machinery while under its influence.

Travel sickness is linked to the vestibular apparatus housed in the inner ear. To conclude this chapter we now discuss this aspect of anatomy and specifically a condition known as Ménière's disease.

The inner ear

The anatomy of the ear can be a little confusing, especially since this organ is responsible not only for hearing but also for balance. There are three components to the ear: the outer ear, the middle ear and the inner ear. All three are involved in hearing but only the inner ear is responsible for balance. It would seem reasonable therefore that we review the inner ear and its role in balance.

The inner ear interprets and transmits sound (auditory) sensations and balance (vestibular) sensations to the brain. It is small (about the size of a pea) and complex in shape and its series of interconnected chambers has been compared to a labyrinth. The main components of the inner ear are the vestibule, the semicircular canals and the cochlea.

The vestibule, a round open space which accesses various passageways, is the central structure within the inner ear. The outer wall of the vestibule contains the oval and round windows (which are the connection sites between the middle and inner ear). Internally, the vestibule contains two membranous sacs, the utricle and the saccule, which are lined with tiny hair cells and attached to nerve fibres, serving as the vestibular (balance/equilibrium) sense organs.

Attached to the utricle within the vestibular portion of the inner ear are three loop-shaped, fluid-filled tubes called the semicircular canals. These are named according to their location ('lateral', 'superior' and 'posterior') and are arranged perpendicularly to one another, like the floor and two corner walls of a box. The semicircular canals are a key part of the vestibular system and allow for maintenance of balance when the head or body rotates. These signals are sent to the brain via a nerve called the auditory or eighth cranial nerve.

Ménière's disease

Ménière's disease is named after the French physician Prosper Ménière and is a rare disorder that affects the inner ear. It can cause vertigo, tinnitus, hearing loss and aural fullness (feeling of pressure in the ear).

The symptoms of Ménière's disease usually appear without warning, although some people complain of a feeling of fullness in one of their ears. The symptoms are often referred to as 'attacks'. Hearing fluctuation or changes in tinnitus may precede an attack. The attacks usually last for around two to three hours, and following an attack it may take one or two days for the symptoms to disappear completely. Following a severe attack, most people find they are exhausted and must sleep for several hours.

A Ménière's attack generally involves severe vertigo (spinning), imbalance, nausea and vomiting. There is a large amount of variability in the duration of symptoms. Some people experience brief 'shocks' while others have constant unsteadi-ness. An unusual sensitivity to visual stimuli is common.

Ménière's disease progresses through different stages. The early stage may consist of between 6 and 11 attacks a year. In the later stages there are usually fewer attacks and they eventually stop. However, hearing loss, tinnitus and balance problems may become constant.

The disease is thought to be caused by fluctuating pressure of the fluid within the inner ear. A system of membranes, called the membranous labyrinth, contains a fluid called endolymph. The membranes can become dilated like a balloon when pressure increases (hydrops).

It is difficult to establish how common Ménière's disease is because the diagnosis criteria tend to vary. However, in the UK it is estimated that around 1 in 1,000 people develop the disease.

Ménière's disease can occur at any age, but it most commonly affects people who are between 40 and 60. It is more common in women than in men, with 30 per cent more women affected. In 5 to 7 per cent of cases there may be a family history of the disease. In 60 to 80 per cent of people with the disease the symptoms will improve and disappear after two to eight years.

Antiemetics used in the management of Ménière's disease

For many people the vertigo caused by the disease can be managed by changes in diet, lifestyle and, when necessary, with medicine. Reductions in salt, caffeine, alcohol, nicotine and stress may be all that is required to dramatically reduce the volume and intensity of attacks and symptoms. Many sufferers report that stress can exacerbate symptoms or even trigger vertigo attacks. It is known that many changes occur in the body when experiencing stress, which no doubt can influence all parts of the body, including the inner ear. For most the number one priority is managing the vertigo, and consequently treatments tend to focus on this.

The inner ear endolymph fluids contain virtually no sodium. Controlling salt in the diet should assist in the regulation of this, preventing swelling (hydrops) in the inner ear and subsequent attacks.

Many doctors will prescribe a diuretic to assist the reduction of fluid retention. For some, medication may also be required to control or reduce the vertigo.

Betahistine

Betahistine is a medicine that closely resembles the natural substance histamine and is used to relieve the symptoms of Ménière's disease. The drug comes as a tablet in either an 8 or 16mg dose. Initially the patient receives a dose of 16mg three times daily; however, as symptoms lessen they will normally be stabilized on a dose of 24–48mg daily. This drug is not recommended for use in children.

Betahistine works by acting on histamine receptors that are found in the walls of blood vessels in the inner ear. By activating these receptors, a process is begun which ultimately reduces the pressure of the fluid that fills the labyrinth in the inner ear. This helps relieve the symptoms associated with Ménière's disease.

Cinnarizine

Cinnarizine works by blocking histamine and muscarinic receptors in the vomiting centre. This prevents the vomiting centre from receiving nerve messages from the vestibular apparatus. In turn, this prevents disturbances in the middle ear from activating the vomiting centre and causing nausea, vertigo and vomiting. The usual dose for an adult is 30mg three times daily. For a child between 5 and 12 years the dose is halved.

Clinical tip

As with other drugs in this class cinnarizine can cause drowsiness and blurred vision. It is important that users make sure their reactions are normal before driving, operating machinery or doing any other jobs which could be dangerous if they are not fully alert or able to see well.

Case studies

① You are a senior student working on a surgical ward. A student from your group has just started their allocation and approaches you. They say they do not understand much about antiemetic drugs and ask you to tell them about cyclizine.

● What is your response?

② A female aged 30 is diagnosed with Ménière's disease and has the accompanying hearing loss and tinnitus. The high-pitched ringing in her ears bothers her. She has now been commenced on betahistine which she hopes will help her condition. The doctor has explained how the drug works, but she did not really understand and asks you to explain again.

● What do you tell her?

Key learning points

Introduction

➢ The major physiological function of emesis (vomiting) is to remove toxic or harmful substances from the body after ingestion.

 →

The vomiting reflex

- The process of emesis can be classified into three phases: nausea, retching and vomiting.
- Mechanoreceptors and chemoreceptors are involved with the detection of emetic stimuli in the GI tract.
- The CTZ acts as the entry point for emetic stimuli.

Management of nausea and vomiting

- Identify and eliminate the underlying cause if possible.
- Control of symptoms if it is not possible to eliminate the underlying cause.

Drug treatment

- Treatments include antihistamines, anticholinergics (block the effects of acetylcholine), dopamine receptor antagonists, 5-HT$_3$ receptor (serotonin) antagonists, cannabinoids, benzodiazepines, corticosteroids and gastroprokinetic agents.

Nausea and vomiting in pregnancy

- The aim in treating nausea and vomiting in pregnancy is to help the woman feel better and to allow them to eat and drink so that they do not become dehydrated or start to lose weight.

Promethazine

- This drug is used to combat moderate to severe morning sickness and hyperemesis gravidarum.
- In the UK promethazine is the drug of first choice.

Prochlorperazine

- Prochlorperazine controls nausea and vomiting by blocking dopamine receptors found in the CTZ.

Metoclopramide

- Metoclopramide is called a 'prokinetic' drug.
- It strengthens the muscle of the lower oesophageal sphincter.

Post-operative nausea and vomiting

- Post-operative nausea and vomiting is detrimental to the patient psychologically and has serious physical consequences.

Ondansetron

- Ondansetron works by blocking the 5-HT$_3$ receptors that are found in the brain and gut.

←

Cyclizine

➢ Directly affects the CTZ by blocking histamine from triggering the vomiting reflex.

Nausea and vomiting in cytotoxic chemotherapy

➢ The acute phase of emesis in chemotherapy responds well to 5-HT_3 antagonists like ondansetron.
➢ Neurokinin (NK_1) receptor antagonists have elicited antiemetic effects in both the acute and especially in the delayed phases of emesis.

Aprepitant

➢ NK_1 receptor antagonist.

Motion sickness

➢ The most common symptoms of motion sickness are dizziness, tiredness and nausea.
➢ The most common theory for the cause of motion sickness is that it functions as a defence mechanism against neurotoxins.

Hyoscine

➢ Hyoscine is one of the best medicines for preventing travel sickness and is derived from plants.

The inner ear

➢ The inner ear is responsible for balance.
➢ The main components of the inner ear are the vestibule, semicircular canals and the cochlea.

Ménière's disease

➢ Thought to be caused by a problem with the pressure in the inner ear.
➢ Most commonly affects people who are between 40 and 60.
➢ A commonly prescribed medication used in the UK is betahistine.

Betahistine

➢ Works by acting on histamine receptors that are found in the walls of blood vessels in the inner ear.

Cinnarizine

➢ Works by blocking histamine and muscarinic receptors in the vomiting centre.
➢ Prevents the vomiting centre from receiving nerve messages from the vestibular apparatus.

Calculations

1   A patient has become dehydrated due to nausea and vomiting. The doctor has prescribed a litre of normal saline to be administered intravenously over an eight-hour period. The giving set delivers 20 drops/ml. How many drops per minute will you set the giving set at?

2   Cyclizine for injection comes as 50mg per ml. However, the doctor only wishes to prescribe 40mg. How much will you draw into the syringe?

3   A doctor prescribes cyclizine 25mg orally. The tablets come as 50mg. How many would you give?

4   Chlorpromazine 25mg is prescribed to be given by IM injection. The stock ampoules contain 50mg in 2ml. How much would you draw up?

5   Metoclopramide 7.5mg is prescribed orally. You have a syrup containing 5mg per 5ml. What dose would you give?

6   Scopolamine 0.25mg has been prescribed. Stock on the placement is 0.4mg in 2ml. How much would you draw up?

7   A child is prescribed metoclopramide 2mg orally. You have been supplied with a syrup containing 5mg in 5ml. How much do you give the child?

8   A child is prescribed promethazine 12.5mg. The tablets come as 25mg. How many do you give to the child?

9   Domperidone is prescribed to a patient at a dosage of 15mg orally three times daily. You have a suspension containing 5mg of the drug in 5ml. How many ml will the patient require in a 24-hour period?

10   A patient is prescribed 48mg of betahistamine orally as a maintenance dose. This dose is to be divided into three equal doses during the day. How many mg does the patient require in each dose?

For further assistance with calculations, please see Meriel Hutton's book *Essential Calculation Skills for Nurses, Midwives and Healthcare Practitioners* (Open University Press 2009).

Multiple choice questions

1 Where is the vomiting centre located?

a) The cerebellum
b) The thalamus
c) The pons
d) The medulla

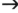

←

2 Which nerve carries excitatory stimuli to the vomiting centre from the gut?

a) Hypoglossal
b) Vagus
c) Trigeminal
d) Abducens

3 What structure acts as the entry point for emetic stimuli and humoral substances?

a) CSF
b) FSH
c) CTZ
d) ADH

4 Which neurotransmitter is *not* linked to inducing vomiting?

a) Gamma-aminobutyric acid
b) Dopamine
c) Histamine
d) Serotonin

5 Which of the following is the preferred antiemetic for use in sickness in pregnancy?

a) Promethazine
b) Ondansetron
c) Metoclopramide
d) Prochlorperazine

6 Ondansetron works by blocking

a) D_4 receptors
b) H_1 receptors
c) $5\text{-}HT_3$ receptors
d) NK_1 receptors

7 Metoclopramide is called a 'prokinetic' drug because it

a) Decreases movement of neurotransmission
b) Works on $5\text{-}HT_3$ receptors
c) Works quicker than other antiemetics
d) Stimulates the muscles of the GI tract

8 Which of the following is the preferred drug for use in Ménière's disease?

a) Metoclopramide
b) Betahistine
c) Ondansetron
d) Prochlorperazine

→

9 Hyoscine is one of the best medicines for preventing

a) Post-operative vomiting
b) Travel sickness
c) Chemotherapy-induced vomiting
d) Morning sickness

10 Aprepitant works by blocking

a) D_4 receptors
b) H_1 receptors
c) $5\text{-}HT_3$ receptors
d) NK_1 receptors

Recommended further reading

Barber, P. and Robertson, D. (2012) *Essentials of Pharmacology for Nurses*, 2nd edn. Maidenhead: Open University Press.

Beckwith, S. and Franklin, P. (2007) *Oxford Handbook of Nurse Prescribing*. Oxford: Oxford University Press.

Bennett, S. (2009) Antiemetics: uses, mode of action and prescribing rationale, *Nurse Prescribing*, 7(2): 63–70.

Brenner, G.M. and Stevens, C.W. (2009) *Pharmacology*, 3rd edn. Philadelphia, PA: Saunders Elsevier.

Clayton, B.D. (2009) *Basic Pharmacology for Nurses*, 15th edn. St Louis, MO: Mosby Elsevier.

Coben, D. and Atere-Roberts, E. (2005) *Calculations for Nursing and Healthcare*, 2nd edn. Basingstoke: Palgrave Macmillan.

Downie, G., Mackenzie, J. and Williams, A. (2007) *Pharmacology and Medicines Management for Nurses*, 4th edn. Edinburgh: Churchill Livingstone.

Gatford, J.D. and Phillips, N. (2006). *Nursing Calculations*, 7th edn. Edinburgh: Churchill Livingstone Elsevier.

Greenstein, B. (2009) *Clinical Pharmacology for Nurses*, 18th edn. Edinburgh: Churchill Livingstone.

Harker, N., Montgomery, A. and Fahey, T. (2004) Treating nausea and vomiting during pregnancy: case progression, *British Medical Journal*, 328(7435): 337.

Heeney, E. (2005) Improving care for patients with nausea and vomiting, *Nursing Times*, 101(14): 33.

Hutton, M. (2009) *Essential Calculation Skills for Nurses, Midwives and Healthcare Practitioners*. Maidenhead: Open University Press.

Karch, A.M. (2008) *Focus on Nursing Pharmacology*, 4th edn. Philadelphia, PA: Lippincott Williams & Wilkins.

Knight, R. (2004) Understanding the aetiology of post-operative nausea & vomiting and reviewing current treatment, *Nurse2Nurse*, 4(3): 12–14.

Lapham, R. and Agar, H. (2009) *Drug Calculations for Nurses: A Step-by-step Approach*, 3rd edn. London: Arnold.

Olver, I. (2004) Aprepitant in antiemetic combinations to prevent chemotherapy-induced nausea and vomiting, *International Journal of Clinical Practice*, 58(2): 201–6.

Peacock, S. (2006) Motion sickness, *Practice Nursing*, 17(1): 25–7.

Simonson, T., Aarbakke, J., Kay, I., Coleman, I., Sinnott, P. and Lyssa, R. (2006) *Illustrated Pharmacology for Nurses*. London: Hodder Arnold.

Starkings, S. and Krause, L. (2010) *Passing Calculation Tests for Nursing Students*. Exeter: Learning Matters.

Zubairi, I. (2006) Management of chemotherapy-induced nausea and vomiting, *British Journal of Hospital Medicine*, 67(8): 410–13.

5

Drugs used in anaesthesia

Learning objectives

After studying this chapter you should be able to:

- Define the term 'anaesthesia'.
- Be aware of the historical development of anaesthetic drugs.
- Understand why no two anaesthetics are the same.
- Outline the safety measures taken prior to anaesthesia.
- Describe the triad and stages of anaesthesia.
- Understand the terms 'induction', 'maintenance' and 'reversal' of anaesthesia.
- Name the intravenous and inhalational anaesthetic agents used, together with the advantages and disadvantages of each.
- Demonstrate knowledge of the mechanisms of how anaesthetic drugs work.
- Provide examples of peri- and post-operative analgesic drugs.
- Explain how muscle relaxants work, the reason for their use and how their effects may be reversed.
- Appreciate the need for adjuvant antiemetic drugs.
- Describe the conduct of a general anaesthetic.

Introduction

The term 'anaesthesia' means 'without sensation'. In practice, this means feeling no pain, something we can expect with modern anaesthesia but this hasn't always been the case. Early surgery was experimental, swift and brutal, carried out as a last resort. It guaranteed a degree of (often excruciating) pain but there was no guarantee of success or asepsis. Alcohol, opium, herbs, poultices and techniques such as cold and nerve compression were employed to minimize pain, with variable effects.

In the nineteenth century, the scope of surgery was limited to the body surface, limbs (amputations), fungating cancers and 'cutting for stone' (lithotomy – the removal of bladder stones). Internal areas such as the chest, abdomen and skull were essentially 'no go'. Speed was essential, and patients were held or strapped down during the ordeal, fainting from agony if they were lucky. Many died during surgery or immediately afterwards. Things were, however, changing. Nitrous oxide, a gas which alters consciousness and provides some pain relief, had been synthesized in the late 1790s. The introduction of ether (by Morton in 1846), and chloroform (by Simpson in 1847) followed. The introduction of ether (and antisepsis through Lister's

carbolic spray in 1865) meant the focus of surgery could be more on accuracy than speed, and surgeons could move into the previously inaccessible areas of the abdomen, chest and brain.

Barbiturate intravenous (IV) induction agents were next to be developed. Thiopentone was first administered in 1934, enabling the patient to become unconscious quickly, smoothly and pleasantly. Muscle relaxant drugs were introduced into anaesthesia in 1942 in the form of d-tubocurarine, based on curare, used by the South American Indians in hunting since the fifteenth century. Over subsequent decades several muscle relaxant drugs were added to the formulary. Halothane, a revolutionary, easy to use, inhalational agent was introduced in the 1950s, remaining popular until the 1980s.

Development and refinement of drugs used in anaesthesia has enabled much safer and far more effective agents to become available, significantly reducing the amount of drugs necessary during the pre-, peri- and post-operative periods, many of which were needed to counteract the unwanted effects of earlier drugs used.

Anaesthesia has developed alongside many social and political influences. Industrial accidents and war injuries have justified anaesthetics being given to people in potentially fatal circumstances, and anaesthetics can now be given to people previously considered unfit. With sophisticated monitoring systems and a greater understanding of the complex way our body functions, anaesthesia is not now confined to surgery. It is required in many situations, carried out by appropriately trained doctors (anaesthetists) in numerous clinical areas. These include operating theatres, intensive care units, A&E, outpatients, dental and GP surgeries, day surgical units, maternity units and chronic pain clinics. Anaesthesia is also used to ease pain at the end of life. Anaesthetic nurses and skilled assistants work together with anaesthetists, providing continuous care to the patient throughout the peri-operative period, ensuring optimal safety and comfort.

Modern anaesthesia

Between 4 and 6 million anaesthetics are carried out annually in the UK. Modern anaesthesia is safe, with a mortality rate of less than 1 in 250,000 directly related to anaesthesia. Patients can expect to be unconscious, pain free, and have no recollection of the surgical procedure. The majority of patients undergo surgery and go home the same day, or even after half a day.

> **Clinical tip**
>
> For many people, especially children, undergoing surgery may be their first and only experience of a hospital environment. Their peri-operative care, from admission to discharge, must be carefully planned by the multidisciplinary team to avoid any distress to the patient and their family.

An anaesthetic can be local, regional or general. Local and regional anaesthesia has been covered by Barber and Robertson (2012). This chapter focuses on general anaesthesia and the pharmacological journey of the patient.

> **Clinical tip**
>
> No two anaesthetics are exactly the same, and each requires adaptation to the individual patient and their clinical circumstances.

The three phases of a general anaesthetic

There are three phases to a general anaesthetic. The first is *induction*. Here, drugs take the patient from wakefulness to a controlled, steady and reversible state of unconsciousness. Surgery will not begin until the anaesthetist is sure the patient is fully and safely anaesthetized. The patient remains in this steady state of anaesthesia throughout the surgical procedure: this is the *maintenance* phase. Once surgery is complete, the anaesthetic is stopped; drugs are withdrawn and, as their effect wears off, the patient returns to *consciousness*. Any drugs having prolonged or detrimental actions will be reversed enabling the patient to return to their fully conscious state.

The safe journey through the three phases of the anaesthetic requires a personalized and balanced regimem of drugs. These are selected from three broad domains or areas, known as the 'triad of anaesthesia', discussed in detail later. First, we must consider how the anaesthetist can be sure the patient is fit for anaesthesia. This is particularly important, as they are unlikely to see the patient again until the day of the anaesthetic.

Prior to anaesthesia

In advance of a planned anaesthetic, a thorough pre-operative assessment is carried out to identify, minimize, eliminate or accommodate any risks. Effective pre-operative assessment can also significantly reduce fear and anxiety, allowing the patient to ask questions. The anaesthetist will use the documented 'core' information to help determine the best combination of drugs and dosages, and the degree of monitoring required to ensure a safe and effective anaesthetic.

Clinical tip

In emergencies a detailed pre-operative assessment may be compromised due to the urgency of the situation, and special measures are taken to ensure safety.

Specialist nurses, working closely with anaesthetists, carry out pre-operative assessments, often in a pre-operative assessment clinic. Patients may be asked to complete a pre-anaesthetic questionnaire and bring it with them.

Clinical tip

Standard pre-operative assessment forms have been produced. National policies are available, and guidelines may be found at the websites of the National Institute for Health and Clinical Excellence (NICE), the National Health Service (NHS) Institute for Innovation and Improvement and the Royal College of Anaesthetists (RCoA). Local policies are also available.

The assessment explores the following:

- history and nature of the presenting condition, the planned operation and the patient's understanding of it;
- medical, surgical and, where relevant, obstetric history, current health status, mental health and disabilities and any other existing conditions;
- family history;
- anaesthetic history, including previous postoperative complications;
- current medications, including prescribed, self-medications and herbal remedies;
- smoking, alcohol intake and other recreational drugs;
- allergies;
- acid reflux.

Clinical tip

It is essential that all relevant information is gathered and recorded with the patient holding nothing back.

Observations and investigations

A number of observations and investigations will be made, depending on circumstance and established local protocols. Blanket routine pre-operative investigations, however, are considered inefficient, expensive and unnecessary. They may even place the patient at risk or delay surgery. Pulse, blood pressure, respiration rate and blood oxygen saturation levels (SaO_2) will be recorded. Other investigations such as chest X-ray, ECG and blood tests (including haemoglobin), liver function tests, urea and electrolytes will be made *only* if indicated.

In addition:

- a physical examination must be undertaken to establish cardiovascular and respiratory integrity;
- swabs will be taken from the nose and groin to identify Methicillin-resistant *Staphylococcus aureus* (MRSA);
- the mouth, teeth and airway are assessed and may be given a 'Mallampati' (or modified version) score or status (l to IV). A high Mallampati score (lll or lV) is associated with a more difficult intubation as well as a higher incidence of difficulty maintaining an airway during the anaesthetic;
- appropriate veins are identified for ease of cannulation;
- accurate documentation of weight, height and body mass index (BMI) are taken to identify underweight or obesity, providing a baseline for some drug calculations;
- impairment of mobility (including the cervical spine and the tempero-mandibular joint which connects the lower jaw to the skull) and rheumatoid associated mobility problems are checked as these may increase the possibility of a more difficult intubation.

The anaesthetist will decide which regular medications should be continued, but in general these include:

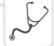

Clinical tip

Some regular medication drugs and herbal remedies need to be stopped prior to surgery. Others need to be continued or modified. National guidelines are available, alongside those determined locally.

The following drugs must be stopped:

- **Warfarin.** This drug should be stopped a number of days before surgery and replaced with low molecular weight heparins such as tinzaparin and enoxaparin. Anticoagulant therapy is carefully managed and monitored into the post-operative period following national and local protocols.
- **Diuretics.** Stopped to avoid a drop in blood volume and potassium depletion. Guidelines are determined locally, but often the morning dose is not given pre-operatively.
- **Oral glucose-lowering drugs.** To prevent hypoglycaemia during surgery. Peri-operative dosing depends on the nature of the operation as well as the severity of diabetes.
- **Some herbal remedies.** For example, echinacea, garlic, ginger, ginkgo biloba, ginseng, St John's wort and valerian (see Chapter 10).

Other concurrent medications needing consideration include monoamine oxidase inhibitors (MAOIs), lithium, oral contraceptives, hormonal replacement therapy and tricyclic antidepressants.

Clinical tip

Most drugs stopped pre-operatively are restarted once oral intake commences. Alternative routes of administration may be required if this is delayed. Some drugs may need modification after surgery.

- **Steroids** to prevent adrenal insufficiency.
- **Opioids** to maintain pain relief and prevent withdrawal symptoms.
- **Anticonvulsants**.
- **Bronchodilators** to prevent bronchoconstriction.
- **Antihypertensives and most cardiovascular drugs** (especially beta blockers) to prevent hypertension and heart problems.
- **Insulin** where the dose will need decreasing as the patient is not eating.
- **Anti-Parkinsonian drugs**.

Once the assessment is complete the anaesthetist will give the patient an ASA (American Society of Anesthesiologists) rating which classifies patients according to their medical status and predicts any potential risk under anaesthesia:

I   Healthy

II Mild systemic disease with no functional impairment

III Moderate systemic disease with functional impairment

IV Severe systemic disease that is a constant threat to life

V   Not expected to survive 24 hours with or without surgery

VI Brain-dead non-heartbeating organ donor

Premedication

A premedication used to be given routinely by intramuscular (IM) injection an hour or so before anaesthesia, but it is not routine practice today to give any premedicant (premed) drugs. However, a premed may sometimes be given, usually orally, to complement and improve the quality of the anaesthetic and the patient experience. The most common reasons are:

- to relax the patient and relieve anxiety (anxiolytic drugs);
- to lessen the incidence of nausea and vomiting (antiemetics);
- to prevent unwanted effects such as excessive upper respiratory tract secretions or bronchospasm (antimuscarinic drugs).

Premedication may also be given to check the pH of gastric secretions and empty the stomach more rapidly, thereby increasing safety.

It is perfectly natural for patients to be apprehensive and anxious prior to a general anaesthetic but this is not usually excessive. However, some patients have specific fears or even phobias. These include embarrassment, loss of control, fear that the wrong operation will be performed, fear that their problem is much worse than expected, fear that they may not wake up after the operation or that they will remain awake during the operation, fear of pain and fear of needles. Others fear talking and embarrassing themselves, giving away personal secrets, or incontinence.

benzodiazepines is covered in Barber and Robertson (2012). Since very few patients are admitted before the day of surgery, these drugs are not usually given on the ward, but may be given in the anaesthetic room, as are antimuscarinic drugs and antiemetics. Analgesic drugs should be continued for patients already in hospital.

The triad of anaesthesia

The triad of anaesthesia (see Figure 5.1) embraces the three basic requirements of an anaesthetic that must be achieved to ensure a successful outcome. The triad is a very convenient way of considering anaesthetic drugs for general anaesthesia because a person will often, although not always, be given drugs from all three areas. A knowledge of which drugs are used for each part of the triad, and why, will help with an overall understanding of the patient experience and subsequent recovery from anaesthesia.

Controlled reversible unconsciousness

You will often see the terms 'hypnosis' or 'narcosis' used to describe this part of the triad. As both terms have other meanings, for accuracy and simplicity

> **Clinical tip**
>
> Observe the patient for verbal and non-verbal signs of anxiety. Being approachable, taking the time to listen and responding appropriately in a clear, simple and friendly manner can go a long way to making the patient less anxious, more reassured, better prepared and therefore more relaxed prior to their anaesthetic. This may also aid their recovery.

One of the benzodiazepines (usually lorazepam or midazolam) is sometimes given to reduce anxiety and provide some amnesia and sedation without having any significant effects on the respiratory or cardiovascular systems. These drugs have a rapid onset and, relative to other benzodiazepines, are short acting. The general use of

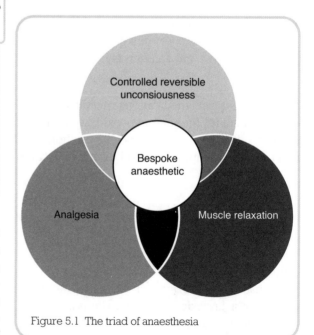

Figure 5.1 The triad of anaesthesia

we describe it here as the induction and maintenance of *controlled reversible unconsciousness*, together with loss of recall of the procedure. A variety of drugs, given intravenously and/or via inhalation are used to do this. The patient journey involves travelling safely from full consciousness to unconsciousness and back to consciousness again.

As the patient becomes unconscious, three observable stages or *planes of anaesthesia* have been identified. These are observed in reverse order as the patient travels back to consciousness again. A fourth, undesirable, stage has also been described.

These stages were first described by Guedel in 1937 when ether was the sole anaesthetic agent used to (relatively slowly) induce unconsciousness. Recognition that patients progressed through the stages helped anaesthetists to control the depth of the anaesthetic. Ether is no longer used in western anaesthesia. However, while quicker-acting modern drugs and techniques 'blur' the observed classical signs of transition from one stage to the next, knowing about the stages is a practical tool in helping us to have an idea of how the anaesthetic is progressing (especially Stage II) and reversing.

Stage I

This begins with the induction of anaesthesia and ends with the patient's loss of consciousness and pain sensation, hence it is called the stage of *analgesia*. Motor activity and reflexes remain normal. This has also been described as the stage of *disorientation*.

Stage II

This extends from the loss of consciousness, through a stage of irregular and spasmodic breathing, to the re-establishment of regular breathing. This stage is called the stage of *(involuntary) excitement* or *delirium*, and is not without danger. There is loss of consciousness, but reflexes are heightened. The patient may swallow, retch, vomit or struggle. (Some may become quite amorous, and some may cry, when returning to consciousness).

Stage III

This is the desired stage of anaesthesia when surgery may begin. It can be subdivided into four planes: light, medium, deep and very deep (too deep). Here, all the reflexes disappear as the stage deepens, and skeletal muscles become relaxed.

Stage IV

This fourth stage must be avoided as it indicates too deep a plane of anaesthesia relative to the amount of surgical stimulation. There is medullary (brainstem) depression and imminent compromise; respiration stops with potential cardiovascular collapse. This stage is reversible if the anaesthetic is lightened and mechanical respiration commenced.

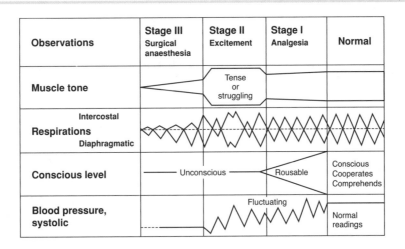

Figure 5.2 Changes in physiological observations during the stages of anaesthesia

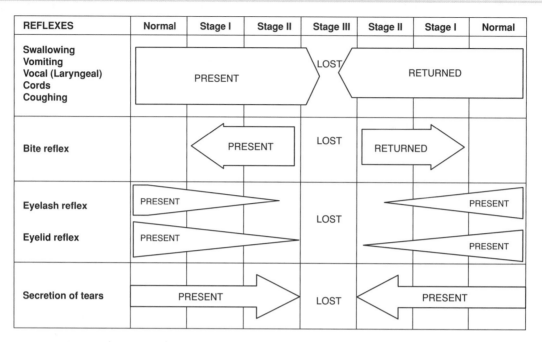

REFLEXES	Normal	Stage I	Stage II	Stage III	Stage II	Stage I	Normal
Swallowing Vomiting Vocal (Laryngeal) Cords Coughing		PRESENT		LOST	RETURNED		
Bite reflex		PRESENT		LOST	RETURNED		
Eyelash reflex	PRESENT			LOST		PRESENT	
Eyelid reflex	PRESENT					PRESENT	
Secretion of tears	PRESENT			LOST	PRESENT		

Figure 5.3 Reflex responses when travelling from consciousness to unconsciousness and back again

Analgesia

This refers to the use of drugs and techniques to ensure the patient recovers with as little pain as possible. These drugs also suppress the physiological reflexes that occur following surgical stimulation. Where intubation is required, analgesia will help to suppress the specific cardiovascular responses occuring as the tube is passed into the trachea. Some analgesia may be administered pre-operatively as well as during the procedure. Post-operative pain is managed through a variety of methods and techniques of administration of analgesia. The specific drugs used are outlined later in the chapter.

The very nature of a surgical procedure necessitates injury to normal healthy tissue. Damaged tissues elicit both local and systemic physiological responses, commensurate with sympathetic stimulation ('fight or flight'). They release chemicals which trigger a local inflammatory response leading to vasospasm, coagulation and the initiation of healing.

Neurological pathways are stimulated, their response being proportionate to the amount of nociceptive stimuli (see Chapter 3 of Barber and Robertson 2012) and tissue injury, along with cardiovascular, respiratory, endocrine, metabolic and inflammatory responses associated with the fight-or-flight mechanism of the autonomic nervous system. Increased sympathetic nervous system activity releases large amounts of adrenal catecholamines (adrenaline and noradrenaline), resulting in increased respiration, blood pressure and heart rate. While these increases can compensate for blood loss as a result of surgery (resulting in a drop in blood volume) they also have detrimental effects. Anaesthetic agents and analgesic drugs work together to reduce the above responses. In

Clinical tip

Pain responses to surgery still occur when the patient is unconscious. Although not 'felt' as pain, the body will still respond to the surgical stimulus. Pain must therefore be reduced as far as possible in both conscious and unconscious states.

turn, this can lessen the cardiovascular risk as well as improving the analgesic outcome.

Muscle relaxation

Often an integral part of modern anaesthesia, *muscle relaxation* refers to the need for a reduction or temporary elimination of muscle tone. (This can still be present when the patient is unconscious.) Relaxants are needed if an endotracheal tube needs to be passed as part of the anaesthetic procedure and also to ensure muscles are sufficiently relaxed to allow the surgeon to access the site of the operation.

> **Clinical tip**
>
> If you rub your abdomen you will find your muscles automatically 'resist' and contract. The same would happen if a surgeon attempted to insert a surgical blade, making surgery extremely difficult, if not impossible, and necessitating first administering a muscle relaxant.

An endotracheal tube is commonly passed into the trachea (known as 'intubation') via the nose or mouth. This maintains an unobstructed, protected airway, both when the patient breathes spontaneously during surgery and when they are artificially ventilated. An inflated cuff around the tube also prevents aspiration of gastric contents. A short-acting neuromuscular blocking agent is generally required to facilitate the passing of the tube, whereas longer-acting drugs are needed for long operations and prolonged artificial ventilation. A detailed account of the long- and short-acting muscle relaxants is given in the next section.

Anaesthetic drugs

A cocktail of drugs selected from the triad is used to provide a balanced individual anaesthetic via two major routes of administration: inhaled (IH) and IV. The optimal combination of agents for any given

Box 5.1 IV and IH agents

IV agents	IH agents
Propofol	Volatile agents: sevoflurane, desflurane, isoflurane
Thiopentone	Enflurane and halothane
Etomidate	Nitrous oxide, oxygen
Ketamine	

patient and procedure is selected by the anaesthetist.

Intravenous anaesthetics (IV)

IV anaesthetics are used mainly for the induction of anaesthesia where they rapidly produce unconsciousness. In most cases their administration is immediately followed with an IH agent or a continued IV infusion to maintain anaesthesia.

Induction with an IV drug is more pleasant for the patient than using an IH agent. This latter takes much longer to induce unconsciousness and involves placing a mask over the face.

> **Clinical tip**
>
> An anaesthetic can be given totally by the IV route. This technique is known as total IV anaesthesia (TIVA) and may be appropriate if volatile agents are not suitable, or there are other particular concerns about their use.

All IV anaesthetic agents are highly lipid soluble, crossing the blood-brain barrier (BBB) effectively and rapidly into the highly vascular brain. The approximate dose of IV anaesthetic drugs is often calculated from body weight.

Clinical tip

Recording the weight of the patient correctly in the pre-operative clinic is essential as the patient is not weighed again prior to receiving drugs calculated by body weight.

The effect of the IV drugs wears off as they are distributed away from the brain to other less well perfused areas. Compared to IH drugs, their offset is very rapid. Unlike IH agents, which are eliminated via the lungs, IV agents are eliminated via the liver or kidneys following biotransformation. IV anaesthetics can cause apnoea as well as dose-dependent depression of cardiac output.

Thiopentone

This is a barbiturate first used in 1930s which, depending on the speed of injection, enables smooth, rapid induction in 10 to 20 seconds and works for approximately five minutes. The termination of action occurs as the drug is redistributed in the blood away from the brain to other tissues, particularly muscle and fat. It is very slowly biotransformed in the liver over several hours. Unlike propofol (see below), it cannot be used as a continuous IV infusion as it would accumulate and lead to prolonged sedation or unconsciousness when discontinued. Adverse effects include vasodilation, respiratory and myocardial depression. Thiopentone has no analgesic effect, in fact it *lowers* the pain threshold (antanalgesia), increasing sensitivity to pain. Thiopentone is also used in critical care to stop seizures and treat elevations in intracranial pressure.

There is usually a period of apnoea after administration, and a dose-dependent drop in blood pressure, mainly due to a decrease in peripheral resistance. Insertion of a laryngeal mask airway following induction with thiopentone requires a neuromuscular blocking (NMB) agent to facilitate insertion and prevent laryngospasm as the laryngeal reflexes are not depressed. The dose is usually between 3 and 5mg/kg, less in the elderly and those suffering from cardiac disease, acidosis or hypovolaemia.

Propofol

Propofol is the most widely used IV agent, and in the 1990s it replaced thiopentone, then the drug of choice. Propofol is a phenol intravenous anaesthetic, chemically unrelated to other anaesthetics. This is formulated in an opaque white emulsion vehicle of soyabean oil and purified egg phosphatide as an IV drug or infusion.

Clinical tip

Egg and soya allergies should be reported to the anaesthetist. Their significance, however, is doubtful.

Depending on the speed of injection, propofol provides rapid unconsciousness (15 to 30 seconds). Its effect lasts for 5 to 10 minutes, followed by a rapid recovery with minimal hangover or cognitive impairment, and low incidence of nausea and vomiting. Unlike thiopentone, it does not cause antanalgesia. When given as a single bolus for induction, its effect is terminated as a result of its being redistributed from the brain to other areas of the body rather than being broken down and metabolized. Maintenance can be achieved either by continuous infusion or intermittent bolus injections, together with either nitrous oxide or opioids to provide analgesia. Infusions of subanaesthetic doses of propofol have been used to sedate patients for surgery under regional anaesthesia, and also to provide sedation of patients in intensive care. Having a shorter offset of action than any other IV induction agent, propofol is particularly useful for outpatient day surgery and short procedures. It is quickly and extensively biotransformed in the liver and therefore doesn't significantly accumulate in the body. It is then excreted, mostly by the kidney. Rapid biotransformation and excretion makes propofol suitable for maintaining anaesthesia with continuous infusion. When used in combination with fentanyl, alfentanil or remifentanil, propofol is suitable for the provision of TIVA. It also has antiemetic properties and does not trigger malignant hyperthermia (see below).

Adverse effects include pain on injection. Administering lignocaine into the vein prior to propofol may lessen this effect. Apnoea on induction occurs more frequently with propofol than with other anaesthetics, and a dose-dependent reduction in ventilation and increase in CO_2 levels occurs when it is used for maintenance of anaesthesia. Convulsions, anaphylaxis and delayed recovery have been reported. Propofol may cause muscle spasm on induction, and occasionally results in green urine. It can significantly decrease blood pressure and heart rate. An NMB is not required when inserting a laryngeal mask airway when propofol is the induction agent.

Because this drug produces a feeling of well-being, its use has occasionally been abused.

Clinical tip

Patients should avoid alcohol, mood-altering drugs, or any other medicines for at least 24 hours after a dose of propofol, unless approved by the prescriber or health care professional.

Dosage of propofol for induction in adults under 55 and children over 12 is 1.5 to 2.5mg/kg at a rate of 20–40mg every 10 seconds until the desired response is achieved. Adults over 55 or debilitated patients receive 1–1.5mg/kg at a rate of 20mg every 10 seconds. The usual dose in children over 8 is 2.5mg/kg but higher doses may be needed in younger children and are administered more slowly. In adults the infusion dose is between 25 and 75mcg/kg per minute to provide sedation and 100 to 200mcg/kg per minute to maintain anaesthesia.

Etomidate

A (methylbenzyl) imidazole derivative, etomidate produces rapid induction of unconsciousness lasting for about 5 to 10 minutes. Full recovery may take longer than with thiopentone. The major advantage of etomidate is that it has little effect on the cardiovascular system and, for this reason, it is sometimes chosen for use in patients with cardiac compromise, and in the elderly. Otherwise, it is not commonly used for induction, or for maintenance of anaesthesia. The induction dose is 0.3mg/kg.

Ketamine

A rapidly acting induction agent, this drug takes 30 to 60 seconds to produce unconsciousness, which lasts for 10 to 15 minutes. As with other IV agents, the effect wears off when it is redistributed in the blood from the brain to other tissues. However, patients may take longer than usual to recover fully. Ketamine is biotransformed by the liver into multiple active metabolites and it has a number of unwanted side-effects.

Ketamine differs from most IV agents because it stimulates the cardiovascular system, resulting in an increased heart rate, blood pressure and cardiac output, causing less hypotension during induction than thiopentone and propofol. This makes it useful for patients with hypovolaemia, and those with cardiac disease/shock as well as children. Respirations are not generally depressed and ketamine causes bronchodilation. Having potent analgesic properties at sub-anaesthetic doses, it can be used for pain relief before a spinal anaesthetic and can be given IV or IM.

Uniquely, ketamine causes a state known as 'dissociative anaesthesia' in which analgesia, amnesia and a dissociation between physiological function and normal communication occurs, resulting in the patient appearing to be awake (with eyes open) but non-communicative. Muscle tone is maintained enabling the patient to maintain their own airway despite being unconscious. During recovery, ketamine can cause 'emergence phenomena': hallucinations, nightmares and psychotic effects. These are so unpleasant in adults (but not children) that it is rarely used and also has a known abuse potential.

The dose via the IV route is 1–2mg/kg, and via the IM route 5–10mg/kg. Lower doses are given to produce sedation, analgesia and amnesia.

Clinical tip

To ensure 'emergence delirium' is kept
to a minimum, noise and stimulation should be
avoided. Patients benefit from recovering in a
quiet part of the recovery room. They may also
benefit from midazolam to minimize disturbing
hallucinations.

Inhalation anaesthetic agents

Anaesthetic drugs administered via this route include several 'volatile agents', oxygen and the gas nitrous oxide. Both vapours and gases are well absorbed by the lungs, which provide a large absorption area (Barber and Robertson 2012) for both topical medicines which act directly on the respiratory system, and for anaesthetic drugs. These are topically applied (by inhalation), absorbed into the bloodstream and circulated to their target tissue (the central nervous system), resulting in suppressed consciousness.

Volatile agents are often referred to as halogenated hydrocarbons or ethers depending on their chemical structure. The term 'halogenated' means that the agent is combined with one of the following chemicals (known as halogens): fluorine, chlorine or bromine. The chemical make-up of the IH anaesthetic agent influences how it works, particularly the speed of onset and offset, and side-effects.

IH drugs include desflurane, sevoflurane, isoflurane and enflurane (halogenated ethers). These have superseded the older halothane (halogenated hydrocarbon) which is now rarely used due to its hepatotoxicity and cardiac instability.

IH agents can be used to induce anaesthesia, although their primary use is to *maintain* the anaesthetic following induction with an IV agent.

Clinical tip

IV drugs such as propofol induce the
anaesthetic rapidly. As their effect wears off (just
a few minutes) an IH agent gradually takes over
to maintain unconsciousness.

Volatile IH agents are supplied in liquid form and at certain temperatures (below room temperature). These liquids give off a gaseous vapour which is administered to patients in precise amounts using calibrated vaporizers and carried in air, oxygen or nitrous oxide oxygen mixtures. They are delivered via a face mask, endotracheal tube or laryngeal mask.

The anaesthetist achieves an individually tailored, precise inspired concentration of IH agent through the use of accurate flow meters and other sophisticated ancillary technology, informed by an in-depth knowledge of the pharmacokinetics and pharmacodynamics of each agent used.

In order to understand the principles of how IH agents exert their effect, you may like to consult Barber and Robertson (2012), Chapter 1, together with the anatomy and physiology of the respiratory and cardiovascular systems.

Key physiological points

- Air is inhaled into the lungs via the nose or mouth, trachea and bronchi before reaching the alveoli of the lungs.
- Oxygen, present in high concentrations in the alveoli, diffuses into nearby capillaries and is transported in the blood, via the heart, to the brain and other vital organs (highly perfused areas) before continuing its journey round the body to supply all the less well perfused tissues.
- Carbon dioxide from the organs and tissues is taken to the lungs in the bloodstream where it crosses over to the alveoli and is exhaled via the lungs, trachea, nose and mouth.

These are important principles because all inhaled anaesthetics enter and leave the body in the same way, through the lungs (Figure 5.4). With each successive breath, more anaesthetic is able to reach the bloodstream. Here it builds up until a therapeutic level of anaesthetic is reached (Stage lll). As long as there is a steady stream of anaesthetic to the brain the patient will remain unconscious. When the concentration of the IH agent becomes equal in the alveoli, blood and

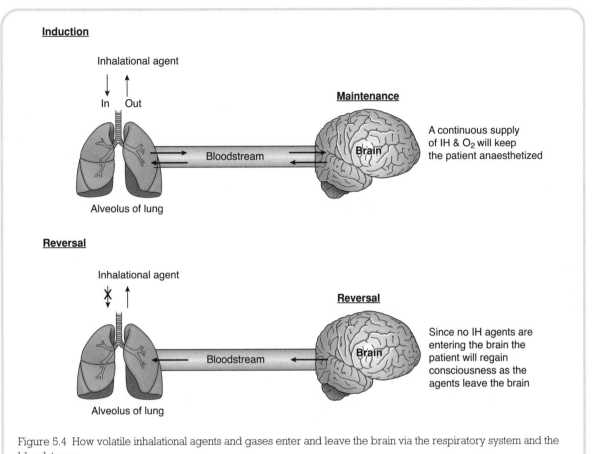

Induction

Inhalational agent

In   Out

Bloodstream

Alveolus of lung

Maintenance

Brain

A continuous supply
of IH & O_2 will keep
the patient anaesthetized

Reversal

Inhalational agent

Bloodstream

Alveolus of lung

Reversal

Brain

Since no IH agents are
entering the brain the
patient will regain
consciousness as the
agents leave the brain

Figure 5.4 How volatile inhalational agents and gases enter and leave the brain via the respiratory system and the bloodstream

brain a steady state of anaesthesia (equilibrium) is reached.

Clinical tip

The patient needs sufficient anaesthetic to maintain Stage III (surgical anaesthesia). If they don't have enough they will return to Stage II and begin to wake up. Too much, and they may enter Stage IV. Remaining at Stage III is achieved by careful monitoring of the patient, and by adjusting the concentration of the anaesthetic agent in the inspired gases.

The perfect IH anaesthetic agent does not exist although modern agents are very safe and relatively trouble free. All the IH agents described be-

low depress the central nervous system and result in unconsciousness, but have no analgesic properties. Potential side-effects of volatile anaesthetics are cardiorespiratory depression, respiratory irritation, hypotension and cardiac arrhythmias (the drugs are *arrhythmogenic*). They can also increase cerebrospinal fluid pressure and therefore should be used cautiously in patients with raised intracranial pressure. Volatile agents can also trigger malignant hyperthermia, a rare inherited condition present in a small number of patients. This results in prolonged muscle contraction and is fatal if not treated with a drug called dantrolene. Volatile inhalational anaesthetics should not be given to patients susceptible to this condition which, if known to be a risk, would have been identified during the pre-operative assessment and an alternative drug such as IV propofol would be used.

Desflurane

Introduced in 1988, desflurane acts rapidly and has a particularly swift emergence rate. It is less potent than isoflurane (see below). It is irritant to the upper respiratory tract, so not recommended for induction since it causes coughing and breath-holding. If administered too rapidly, laryngospasm and increased secretions can occur. Desflurane requires a special vaporizer for administration.

Sevoflurane

Introduced in 1971, this is a very popular (if expensive) potent IH agent with a rapid onset and offset. It is non-irritant and therefore can be used for induction, causing less effect on heart rhythm when compared to other agents. It is particularly suitable for inducing an anaesthetic in children. Sevoflurane is said to be the closest we have to the 'ideal' inhalational anaesthetic.

Isoflurane

Introduced in 1970, this is a popular 'fast-acting' agent which is cheaper than sevoflurane. Isoflurane can irritate mucous membranes, causing cough, breath-holding and laryngospasm.

Enflurane

First used in 1966, this has been superseded by more modern and less toxic agents.

Halothane

This the oldest of the halogenated hydrocarbon drugs (dating from 1956), halothane is rarely used as it has been known to cause liver problems, particularly after repeated exposure within a short time interval. It is a potent agent, with a slower onset and offset of action than any of the above. It may occasionally be used for cardiorespiratory depression, arrhythmias, asthma and when uterine atony is a problem in maternity.

Inhalational gases

These include nitrous oxide and oxygen. Nitrous oxide is a weak (non-halogenated) inorganic anaesthetic gas, stored as a liquid in blue cylinders. It produces a fast-acting, light anaesthetic with a rapid offset, typically administered in a concentration of 70 per cent in oxygen combined with a volatile IH agent. It cannot be used for general anaesthesia on its own, and some anaesthetists do not use it at all.

A major benefit of nitrous oxide is its analgesic properties in concentrations less than those needed to produce unconsciousness (subanaesthetic concentrations), making it ideal for use during labour. Since it is weak, only a certain amount can be administered and it cannot provide general anaesthesia when given as the sole agent. It reduces the amount of other IH agents needed when combined with them.

Side-effects include nausea, vomiting, depression, adverse effects on pregnancy and more serious effects on bone marrow.

Entonox

This is a mixture of oxygen and nitrous oxide in equal (50:50) proportions. Stored as a gas in blue and white cylinders, it is used for pain relief in labour and by ambulance crews for pain relief as a result of injuries.

Oxygen

Although not strictly an anaesthetic agent, oxygen (considered a drug which has to be prescribed) is always included as part of the anaesthetic gas mixture in higher concentrations than those present in air. Patients are often given extra oxygen during induction, a continuous supply during maintenance and high concentrations during the immediate post-operative period.

> **Clinical tip**
>
> IH anaesthetic gases pose an occupational threat. In the past they were freely exhaled into the air of the operating theatre and were associated with higher incidences of spontaneous abortion. 'Scavenging' or removal of waste gases in operating rooms is now routine, and has reduced the concerns of occupational exposure.

Properties of inhalational agents influencing uptake

Potency

IH agents are administered by concentration rather than dose, as it is impossible to measure exactly the amount of drug in the brain. The anaesthetist needs to know how potent the drug is and this is determined by its minimum alveolar concentration or MAC value (described below), how soluble it is in the blood (influencing its speed of uptake) and how soluble the agent is in (fat) oil which will influence the rate at which its effect wears off.

MAC value

The MAC value is worked out by establishing how much of the IH agent needs to be present in the exhaled breath to prevent a response to a skin incision in 50 per cent of subjects. Alternatively, MAC can be calculated using the end-expiratory concentration of a particular IH agent which prevents movement in response to a surgical skin incision in 50 per cent of subjects. If an inhaled anaesthetic is given in a concentration of $1.3 \times$ its MAC value, then it will prevent a response in 95 per cent of subjects. This serves as a guide to the anaesthetist, who will administer and monitor the amount of inspired and expired gas for a particular agent. MAC values are given in Box 5.2.

Blood/gas solubility

The anaesthetic effect is only achieved when the concentration of an IH agent is the same in the blood as it is in the alveoli. A steady state is maintained when the same amount of molecules of anaesthetic enter and leave the blood in a given time. This is primarily determined by the drug's relative solubility in blood and is known as the blood/gas partition coefficient. The less an IH agent dissolves in the blood, the quicker it will build up and diffuse into the central nervous system to suppress consciousness. The more soluble the drug, the more molecules will dissolve in the blood, and the longer it will take for the patient to become anaesthetized.

For example, N_2O has a low blood/gas coefficient of 0.47, as it is hardly soluble in blood at all so acts rapidly. Halothane, however, is very soluble in blood, with a high blood/gas coefficient of 2.3, and therefore takes much longer to get into the central nervous system.

Oil/gas solubility

IH anaesthetics are highly lipid soluble and their degree of lipid solubility is expressed as the oil/gas partition coefficient. We have already seen that IH drugs are taken to the brain in the blood. When the blood containing the anaesthetic leaves the brain, the effect will wear off unless more anaesthetic (present in the blood) is delivered to the brain. This is why a constant supply of IH agent is needed. After it leaves the brain, most of the drug is eliminated by the lungs. A certain amount, however, is absorbed into the body fat, and the longer the anaesthetic the more will be absorbed.

The less soluble the anaesthetic stored in fat (low blood/oil coefficient), the quicker the offset will be and the sooner the patient will wake up. Agents with a high coefficient will delay the return to consciousness.

Biotransformation

It used to thought that IH agents were exhaled unchanged. However, we now know that they are metabolized to a certain extent.

> **Clinical tip**
>
> A low blood/gas coefficient and high MAC value correlate with a rapid onset of induction.

How anaesthetic drugs exert their effects

The precise way anaesthetic drugs work at a molecular level is uncertain. Several possibilities have been suggested, but it is clear that much more research remains to be done before the mechanism of action of anaesthetic drugs is fully known.

Box 5.2 Properties of IH agents

	N₂O	Halothane	Isoflurane	Sevoflurane	Desflurane
MAC*	>105%	0.75%	1.2%	3.3% in neonates to to 1.7 in aduts and 1.5 in the elderly	6%
Onset/offset	Most rapid	Slow	Medium	Rapid	Very rapid
Blood/gas coefficient	0.47	2.3	1.4	0.6	0.4
Respiratory irritation during induction	Low	Low	Moderate	Low	High
Respiratory depression	None	Low	Moderate	Low	Low
Heart rate		Decreased	Increased	Increased	Increased
Blood pressure	None	Decreased	Decreased	Decreased	Decreased
Degree of muscle relaxation	None	Low	Medium	Medium	Medium
Degree of analgesia	Good	None	None	None	None
Arrhythmogenic?	No	High	Low	Low	Low
Amount biotransformed		20%	0.2%	2% to fluoride	0.02%
Cost	Low	Low	High	Very High	Very high

*1 × MAC will prevent a response (movement) to a skin incision in 50 per cent of patients. 1.3 × MAC will prevent a response (movement) to a skin incision in 95 per cent of patients. Note that the MAC value for sevoflurane is slightly lower in children than in adults.

Most theories suggest that the drugs reversibly interact with the hydrophobic (lipid) component of the membrane of the nerve cells (neurons) in the central nervous system. This causes an alteration in the normal 'firing of a neuron' and release of neurotransmitters, slowing the whole process of nerve transmission down, especially in the thalamus, cerebral cortex and spinal cord. It has been suggested that the nerves then take longer to repolarize than normal, resulting in loss of consciousness.

The most likely target is thought to be the ion channels responsible for conduction of the nerve impulse. Anaesthetic drugs may affect the nerve membrane in such a way that Na⁺ and Ca⁺ cannot enter, preventing the nerve from depolarizing. IH and IV anaesthetic agents are known to work at the gamma-aminobutyric acid (GABA) and N-methyl D-aspartate (NMDA) receptors. GABA is a neuro-transmitter which slows (inhibits) brain function (Barber and Robertson 2012). Some anaesthetic agents promote the effect of GABA which opens

Cl⁻ channels. This, in turn, inhibits the response of the neuron to a stimulus by making the inside of the neuron more negative in relation to the outside. IH anaesthetic drugs such as thiopentone, etomidate, benzodiazepines and propofol are thought to bind to the Cl⁻ channel complex and exert their effects in this way. Ketamine blocks the channel of the N-NMDA receptor. The actions of the inhaled agents include increased inhibition via K⁺ channel leakage.

Intra-operative analgesia

An effective anaesthetic requires effective analgesia. Analgesic drugs may be required before, during and after anaesthesia, regardless of whether the patient is awake.

Non-steroidal anti-inflammatory drugs (NSAIDs) are useful as adjuncts to opiates since they do not cause respiratory depression, impair gastrointestinal (GI) motility or cause dependence. Paracetamol, parecoxib, ketolorac and ibrupofen may all be used for analgesia.

Small amounts of rapid acting opiates frequently form an integral part of the induction phase of the anaesthetic. This reduces the amount of anaesthetic drugs needed (known as a 'hypnotic sparing effect'), as well as providing intra-operative analgesia and reducing the physiological responses to surgery. Barber and Robertson (2012) covers analgesic drugs, including the use and unwanted effects of NSAIDs and the opioids morphine and codeine.

Morphine, alfentanil, fentanyl and remifentanil

Morphine is regularly used both intra- and post-operatively. Synthetic opioids (e.g. alfentanil, fentanyl and remifentanil) are commonly used. They act rapidly, within one to two minutes, and have a short duration of action. Fentanyl and alfentanil are short-acting, remifentanil is ultra-short acting. Alfentanil provides analgesia and enhances anaesthesia in short procedures. The dose for induction is 50 to 150mcg/kg IV and 0.1 to 3mcg/kg/min by infusion. Breastfeeding should be withheld for

24 hours following administration. When compared to fentanyl, alfentanil has a slightly faster onset of action, but its effects last only for 5 to 10 minutes following a bolus dose.

Fentanyl is a potent opioid agonist used to provide intra-operative analgesia and enhance anaesthetic drugs. An IV dose of 30mcg/kg will aid the induction of anaesthesia within 30 seconds and last for 30 to 60 minutes. Large doses may last several hours. Fentanyl is useful in cardiovascular anaesthesia as cardiovascular stability remains even after large doses.

Remifentanil is an opiate analgesic available as an infusion only for peri-operative analgesia. Dosage for induction is 0.5 to 1mcg/kg/min; maintenance is 0.05 to 0.08mcg/kg/min. It has a rapid onset of action (similar to alfentanil) with an ultra-short duration of action of three minutes.

Clinical tip

To avoid excessive doses in obese patients the dose of alfentanil, fentanyl and remifentanil may need to be calculated on the basis of *ideal* body weight. Repeated intra-operative doses of alfentanil or fentanyl are given with care, as they may cause respiratory depression which persists into the post-operative period. If this happens the opioid anatagonist naloxone may be used as an antidote.

Adjuvant drugs

Historically the use of adjuvant drugs in anaesthesia has been necessary to counteract the unwanted effects of the anaesthetic agents of the time. Modern drugs such as propofol (IV) and sevoflurane (IH) do not normally cause significant unwanted effects. Measures to minimize the possibility of patients being sick, however, are taken. Nausea and vomiting can be troublesome following anaesthesia, and may even delay discharge. Other adjuvant drugs are administered according to circumstance and patient requirements.

Antiemetics

Drugs that are used in the prevention and control of post-operative nausea and vomiting include: histamine H_1-receptor antagonists; cyclizine; promethazine; 5-HT$_3$ receptor antagonists; ondansetron; granisetron; corticosteroids; dexamethosone (which also reduces swelling); and dopamine D2-receptor antagonists such as metaclopromide and droperidol.

Muscle relaxant drugs (NMBs)

Although anaesthetic agents cause muscle relaxation to a certain extent, this is often insufficient for surgery or intubation; huge doses would be needed to do this. The use of an NMB agent, directly blocking the neuromuscular conduction at the motor end plate, reduces the maintenance dose of anaesthetic agents needed, as well as relaxing all the skeletal and smooth muscles.

Clinical tip

Artificial ventilation is required when using muscle relaxants as they affect *all* muscles, notably those used for respiration.

Depolarizing and non-depolarizing agents

There are two groups of NMB agents: depolarizing and non-depolarizing. Each has a different physiological action and is used in different circumstances. In order to understand how both groups work, we need to look more closely at the chain of events at the *neuromuscular junction* (see Figure 5.5).

Contraction of skeletal muscle is controlled by motor nerves (neurones) that release a chemical neurotransmitter, acetylcholine, into the synapse (gap) where the nerve and muscle meet. This is called the neuromuscular junction. The electrical stimulus (carried by the motor nerve) telling the muscle fibre to contract is carried across the

synapse by acetylcholine. When this meets with the muscle fibre, it attaches to nicotinic acetylcholine receptors on the muscle membrane, causing the opening of ion channels and resulting in the contraction of the muscle fibre. Once the acetylcholine has carried the stimulus for muscle contraction across the gap between the nerve and the muscle it is broken down by the enzyme acetylcholinesterase and returned to the nerve, ready to take more acetylcholine across the neuromuscular junction the next time the muscle fibre needs to contract.

The only depolarizing NMB used in the UK is suxamethonium, which first causes the muscle cells to depolarize (fire). Attaching directly to the acetylcholine receptors on the motor end plate of voluntary muscles, it then prevents the muscle fibres from repolarizing, making them unable to respond to further nerve stimulation while the drug remains attached.

Non-depolarizing NMB agents exert their effect without first depolarizing the muscle fibres. They are known as 'competitive NMBs' because they successfully 'compete' with acetylcholine at the motor end plate nicotinic receptors, forming a barrier which renders the acetylcholine unable to cause the muscle fibre to contract. There are two main groups, the benzylisoqueliniums, including atracurium, cisatracurium and mivacurium, and the aminosteroids which include pancuronium, vecuronium and rocuronium. Some of the former are associated with histamine release which can cause skin flushing, increased heart rate and a drop in blood pressure. The latter are said to produce fewer cardiovascular side-effects.

Clinical tip

NMB agents block the receptors in skeletal muscle, but not in autonomic ganglia. This means that they have little effect on the sympathetic and parasympathetic nervous systems, since the muscarinic receptors are not affected.

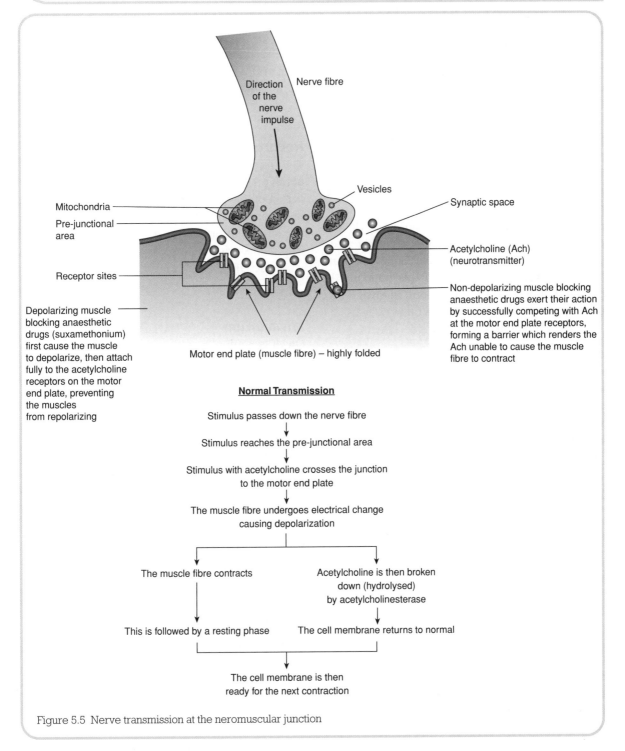

Figure 5.5 Nerve transmission at the neromuscular junction

Suxamethonium

Suxamethonium is also known as Scoline (its proprietary name) and is used predominantly when a rapid onset of muscle relaxation is required. It can also be used in a Caesarian section as it does not cross the placenta.

Suxemethonium is short-acting and the normal intubation dose of 1–1.5mg/kg IV results in full muscle paralysis after 60 seconds, lasting for two to five minutes until the drug is biotransformed by an enzyme in the plasma, (pseudo)cholinesterase. Repolarization then occurs, reactivating the muscle. Abnormalities of plasma cholinesterase can lead to prolonged action and the patient will experience a condition called 'Scoline apnoea'. There is no antidote to suxamethonium, so if this happens the patient will need to be intubated in intensive care until the effect eventually wears off.

Suxamethonium has several side-effects:

- flushing of the skin;
- excessive salivation;
- bradycardia (pronounced with multiple doses);
- post-operative muscle pain;
- prolonged respiratory depression;
- raised intracranial, intra-ocular and intra-abdominal pressure.

> ### Clinical tip
>
>
> Fit young adults in particular may complain of pain and tenderness in their muscles approximately 24 hours after receiving suxamethonium.

Atracurium

Onset is two to three minutes with an intermediate duration of around 20 minutes. It may cause histamine release. It breaks down spontaneously under the influence of body temperature and pH rather than by an enzyme system (Hofmann degradation).

Vecuronium

This drug has an intermediate duration of 20–40 minutes and has little effect on the heart.

Cisatracurium

This is a purified mixture of one isomer of atracurium and behaves very similarly to atracurium, with a slightly lower incidence of flushing and histamine effects.

Rocuronium

This has the fastest onset of action of all competitive NMBs (1–1.5 minutes) and a duration of action of 20–40 minutes. It is occasionally used in high doses as an alternative to suxamethonium. It is excreted in urine and so is not suitable for use in patients with impaired renal function. It has a vagolytic effect which may lead to tachycardia.

Mivacurium

Onset is 3 minutes with a short duration of 15–25 minutes. This drug is associated with considerable histamine release and is metabolized by pseudo-cholinesterase.

Pancuronium

This is an older drug with an onset of 3 minutes and a long duration of action (60–90 minutes). It is not suitable for use in patients with impaired renal function as it is excreted in the urine. Sometimes used in long procedures, it has a vagolytic effect.

> ### Clinical tip
>
>
> Because muscle relaxant drugs relax all the voluntary muscles, including those required for respiration, communication and speech, great care is taken to ensure the patient is maintained in Stage III of unconsciousness. If the patient were to 'lighten' to Stage II or I they would be awake and in pain but unable to move or convey this. Therefore the patient's level of unconsciousness is continuously monitored to prevent 'anaesthetic awareness'.

Reversal of non-depolarizing NMBs

Non-depolarizing NMBs may wear off spontaneously and their effect can quickly be reversed using anticholinesterase drugs. These increase the amount of acetylcholine at the motor end plate, overcoming the barrier created by the non-depolarizing NMB. They act by inhibiting the enzyme acetylcholinesterase which breaks down acetylcholine.

Neostigmine

This is an anticholinesterase specifically used for the reversal of non-depolarizing NMBs. The usual dose of 2.5–5mg acts within 6 minutes of IV injection and its effects last for 20–30 minutes (a second dose may then be necessary). Increasing acetylcholine results in:

- increased mucous production;
- bradycardia;
- blurred vision;
- bronchospasm;
- increased gut motility;
- sweating.

Atropine (1.2mg) or glycopyrrolate (0.5mg) are given with neostigmine to prevent these unwanted side-effects.

Clinical tip

Sometimes the reversal effect of neostigmine wears off before the non-depolarizing NMB, and the patient becomes paralysed again. This is known as *recurarization* and requires immediate intervention.

The conduct of a general anaesthetic

Fasting

An empty stomach is advisable prior to surgery, and is achieved by fasting for several hours. The duration of this period has received considerable attention from the medical and nursing professions, resulting in the production of national guidelines such as those issued by the Royal College of Nursing (RCN), which have been endorsed by the RCoA, the Association of Paediatric Anaesthetists of Great Britain and Ireland, the Royal College of Midwives, the Preoperative Association and the British Association of Day Surgery. Local policies will also dictate practice.

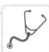

Clinical tip

Under normal circumstances, the longer one doesn't eat, the emptier the stomach will be. However, in certain circumstances (e.g. labour and shock), the stomach does not empty, posing an aspiration risk under anaesthesia.

For children undergoing elective surgery, preoperative fasting is guided by what is known as the '2-4-6 rule', whereby the following fluids may be taken before induction of anaesthesia:

- water and other clear (non-carbonated) fluid: up to **two** hours before;
- breast milk up to **four** hours before;
- formula milk, cow's milk or solids up to **six** hours before.

For adults we apply the '2 and 6 rule':

- clear fluids up to **two** hours before induction;
- minimum pre-operative fasting time of **six** hours for food (solids, milk and milk-containing drinks).

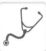

Clinical tip

Be aware of patients who are being fasted for longer periods than recommended and of your local policy. Seriously ill or elderly patients, children, breastfeeding mothers and those who have undergone bowel preparation must not be fasted for long periods of time. They may require IV fluids prior to surgery. Also note that chewing gum constitutes a clear fluid.

Consent

Obtaining informed consent for surgery and anaesthesia is a fundamental part of clinical risk management. This must be correctly signed and dated. The patient should give 'informed written consent' to both the surgical team (for surgery) and the conducting anaesthetist (for the anaesthetic) prior to surgery. It is important that the patient understands the options available, and their attendant benefits and risks, before giving this consent. Once this understanding is manifest, and not before, the consent form is signed and dated. 'Understanding' is the key word here: it is not sufficient that the patient happily signs any paperwork with which they are presented.

Clinical tip

Patients unable to give consent for any reason require special consideration.

Pre-induction

Wherever possible, patients walk to theatre. In the anaesthetic room an IV cannula will be inserted and any monitoring equipment applied. An IV infusion may commence.

Clinical tip

Before coming to theatre, children will often have a local anaesthetic cream applied as a patch to the dorsum of both hands, producing surface anaesthesia prior to cannulation.

A benzodiazepine or short-acting opiate may be given immediately prior to induction of anaesthesia, sedating the patient and providing analgesia. Patients who are at high risk of gastric reflux and aspiration may receive sodium citrate. All patients are given oxygen pre-induction, providing a degree of oxygenation in the functional residual capacity and allowing more leniency with speed of securing the airway.

Induction

This is usually achieved with an IV anaesthetic drug (most commonly propofol). Remember IV agents are short-acting, therefore a volatile inhalational agent, mixed with air, oxygen or nitrous oxide, is needed to maintain the anaesthetic. An NMB agent will be given if muscle relaxation is required for the surgical procedure or prior to intubation.

It is possible to induce an anaesthetic without an IV drug, relying solely on IH. This is unusual, and potentially unpleasant. IV induction is preferred by most adults. IH induction is still commonly used with children if access to a vein is limited due to poor patient cooperation. It may be indicated in adults who have incipient airway obstruction, or those with malignant hyperthermia.

Clinical tip

It takes longer for an anaesthetic to reach high concentrations in a baby than it does in the the mother. This gives a small safety margin allowing the mother to be anaesthetized during the final stages of childbirth.

Airway management

Safe induction involves careful airway control. Depending on circumstances a face mask, laryngeal mask, endotracheal or nasal tube may be used. The airway technique determines the selection of anaesthetic, in turn affecting control of the airway and ventilation. Patients may continue to breathe spontaneously (by themselves) or they can be artificially (mechanically) ventilated.

Laryngospasm

Here, the muscles in the larynx go into spasm as a result of noxious stimuli. Laryngospasm is a dangerous complication of anaesthesia, particularly in Stage ll. The commonest cause of airway obstruction, laryngospasm is often associated with airway manipulation (e.g. intubation or the presence of secretions or blood).

An oropharyngeal airway and a laryngeal mask produce the least stimulation, endotracheal tubes the most. Higher doses of IV anaesthetic and opioids are needed for induction involving tracheal intubation which generally requires the use of NMBs.

Maintenance

The patient is maintained in a balanced plane of anaesthesia by adjusting the IV or inhaled agent, analgesic and muscle relaxation drugs accordingly, and carefully and continuously monitoring the patieint to avoid under- or overdosing. Fluid replacement is maintained.

> **Clinical tip**
>
> The Association of Anaesthetists of Great Britain and Ireland has published guidelines for minimal monitoring during the maintenance of anaesthesia. These are pulse, non-invasive measurement of blood pressure, ECG, O_2 sats, IH gas monitoring and end tidal CO_2.

> **Clinical tip**
>
> Some patients, even those undergoing the same procedure, require more or less anaesthetic than others, affecting their speed of recovery. Age, degree of surgical stimulus and pain, and condition of the patient are some of the reasons for this.

Emergence

On completion of surgery the anaesthetist will:

- switch off the volatile anaesthetic agents and gases;
- continue with analgesia and oxygen, titrated to effect;
- reverse any residual NMB effect.

As the patient travels through the stages of anaesthesia in reverse order and enters Stage ll (excitement) it is important to treat breath-holding, laryngospasm, vomiting and shivering if they occur. It is usual (unless contraindicated), either in theatre or recovery, to give paracetamol (1000mg) in an IV infusion. Oxygen will also be given and titrated to the patient's oxygen saturation.

Recovery

Patients are usually cared for in a specially equipped recovery room, returning to the ward area when sufficiently recovered from the anaesthetic and as pain free as possible. A care plan is put in place for post-operative pain relief and relief of post-operative nausea and vomiting. A wide range of drugs and techniques are available, and national and local policies apply. Pain from minor surgical procedures may be alleviated with paracetamol or other NSAIDs. Moderate pain requires stronger analgesia such as mild opiates (e.g. tramadol, codeine). Major surgical procedures may require a combination of drugs and techniques, including a strong opiate such as morphine delivered by patient-controlled analgesia; epidural analgesia and wound infiltration. Opiates may induce side-effects, including respiratory euphoria, depression, depression of the coughing reflex, nausea, vomiting, reduction of smooth muscle contraction and cardiovascular depression.

After minor surgery and prior to discharge, post-operative care will be continued on the ward. Patients undergoing major surgery may be cared for until well enough to be discharged, others may require intensive care or high dependency care.

Miscellaneous drugs kept in recovery

> **Clinical tip**
>
> A number of drugs are kept in recovery for emergency use and for the management of post-operative pain and associated side-effects of anaesthesia. All emergency and necessary monitoring equipment is to hand.

The following drugs will normally be found in the recovery area:

- naloxone (reverses actions of opiates);
- doxapram (a direct respiratory stimulant);
- glycopyrronium bromide (reverses brady-cardia);
- ketolorac (an NSAID);
- midazolam (a benzodiazepine sedative);
- flumazenil (reverses benzodiazepines);
- oxycodone (a strong opiate);
- fentanyl (a strong opiate);
- antiemetics;

- dantrolene (for the treatment of malignant hyperthermia);
- suggamadex (for emergency reversal of rocuronium-induced NMB).

Clinical tip

Although anaesthetic techniques are similar across the age continuum, drug dosage will vary enormously. Elderly or debilitated patients, at greater risk of an adverse outcome, need special consideration. Anaesthetic requirement may be less than in healthy adults.

Case studies

① Hamza Munir is 4 years old, weighs 15kg and is about to undergo day case surgery to remove adenoids and tonsils. He arrives in the anaesthetic room with patches of local anaesthetic cream on the dorsum of each hand. Once a 22g cannula is inserted, Hamza receives propofol 60mg IV (4mg/kg) followed by IH sevoflurane carried in O_2 and air. An endotracheal tube is passed, with use of atracurium. He receives dexamethasone 3.8mg and ondansetron 1.5mg IV; paracetamol 300mg; diclofenac 2.3mg and morphine 1.5mg (via suppository). An infusion of saline 150ml is administered. At the end of the surgery his residual NMB is reversed with a neostigmine/glycopyrrolate mixture.

- Why would Hamza have local anaesthetic 'patches' on each hand?
- With reference to the triad of anaesthesia, which of the above drugs were used to induce and maintain unconsciousness, and which were to provide analgesia?
- Which drugs are antiemetics? Why is their administration so important intra-operatively?

② Abbi Rooney is 39 years old, 1.6m tall and weighs 74kg. Scheduled to undergo a hysterectomy due to endometriosis, she is otherwise fit, with no allergies. Prior to induction of anaesthesia she is given fentanyl 100mcg IV, propofol 200mg IV followed by isoflurane carried in O_2 and air. A variety of antiemetic and analgesic drugs are also administered and topped up during the anaesthetic. Rocuronium 50mg is administered prior to an oral, cuffed endotracheal tube being passed. At the end of the operation glycopyrronium bromide 0.5mg and neostigmine 2.5mg are used to reverse the muscle relaxant.

- Why was Abbi given fentanyl prior to induction?
- Why was an endotracheal tube required?
- How does the NMB agent rocuronium work?
- Why are glycopyrronium bromide and neostigmine required to reverse the effects of rocuronium?

Key learning points

Introduction

➤ Anaesthesia means 'without sensation'; an anaesthetic can be local, regional or general. Anaesthesia is not confined to surgery but is required in many situations.

Modern anaesthesia

➤ Modern anaesthesia is safe. Patients can expect to be unconscious, pain free and with no recollection of the surgical procedure.
➤ The majority of patients undergoing surgery return home the same day (sometimes after half a day).

The three phases of a general anaesthetic

➤ Induction.
➤ Maintenance.
➤ Emergence.

Prior to anaesthesia

➤ A pre-operative assessment is carried out to identify, minimize, eliminate or accommodate any risks.
➤ A number of observations and investigations are made. Blanket, routine pre-operative investigations should not be carried out.
➤ Some routine medications must be stopped, some continued, others modified.
➤ Pre-medicant drugs are occasionally given to complement and improve both the quality of the anaesthetic and the patient experience.

The triad of anaesthesia

➤ The three domains of anaesthesia (unconsciousness, analgesia, muscle relaxation) are called the triad of anaesthesia.
➤ Three observable stages or planes of anaesthesia have been identified. A fourth, undesirable, stage has also been described.

Anaesthetic drugs

➤ A variety of IV and volatile IH drugs, mixed with air, oxygen or nitrous oxide, are used to induce and maintain unconsciousness.
➤ Analgesic drugs may be given before, during and after anaesthesia, keeping the patient as pain free as possible.
➤ Muscle relaxant drugs are often used when the patient is intubated for long procedures or when muscles are cut during surgery.

➤ Antiemetics are given as adjuvants, preventing post-operative nausea and vomiting.
➤ Other drugs are given as required.

The conduct of a general anaesthetic

➤ Fasting is required to ensure the stomach is empty, minimizing risk of aspiration.
➤ Informed consent to anaesthesia is essential.
➤ The anaesthetic room is prepared, the patient comfortably and safely positioned and an IV cannula inserted.
➤ Induction usually takes place via an IV drug followed by an IH agent in air. Analgesic drugs and an NMB will be given if required.
➤ Safe induction involves careful airway management.
➤ IV or inhaled agent, analgesia and muscle relaxation drugs are adjusted accordingly. The patient is carefully and continuously monitored to avoid underdosing and overdosing. Fluid replacement will be maintained.
➤ For emergence the administration of anaesthetic drugs is stopped and any residual effects terminated. Analgesia and O_2 are continued. Airway management in Stage ll is closely observed.
➤ Patients are usually cared for in a specially equipped recovery room, returning to the ward area when sufficiently recovered from anaesthetic and as free from pain as possible.

Multiple choice questions

1 The term 'anaesthesia' means

a) Without pain
b) Without sensation
c) Without consciousness
d) All of the above

2 A high Mallampati score is associated with

a) High blood pressure
b) MRSA
c) A difficult intubation
d) A high temperature

3 How many phases are involved in administering an anaesthetic?

a) 1
b) 2
c) 3
d) 4

4 Which of the following routine medications need to be stopped prior to anaesthesia?

a) Warfarin
b) Diuretics
c) Oral glucose-lowering drugs
d) Herbal remedies

5 Which or the following should continue to be taken?

a) Herbal remedies
b) Steroids
c) Warfarin
d) Anticonvulsants

6 Which of the following is not an IH agent?

a) Nitrous oxide
b) Sevoflurane
c) Propofol
d) Isoflurane

7 How is the concentration of an IH agent calculated?

a) By the patient's weight
b) By its MAC value
c) In ml
d) In mcg

8 The most popular IV anaesthetic agent is

a) Thiopentone
b) Aracurium
c) Halothane
d) Propofol

9 A drug with a high blood/gas coefficient will

a) Act rapidly
b) Wear off rapidly
c) Take a long time to act
d) Take a long time to wear off

10 Which of the following muscle relaxants is a depolarizing agent?

a) Atracurium
b) Suxamethonium
c) Pancuronium
d) Rocuronium

Recommended further reading

Barber, P. and Robertson, D. (2012) *Essentials of Pharmacology for Nurses*, 2nd edn. Maidenhead: Open University Press.

Beckwith, S. and Franklin, P. (2007) *Oxford Handbook of Nurse Prescribing*. Oxford: Oxford University Press.

Brenner, G.M. and Stevens, C.W. (2009) *Pharmacology*, 3rd edn. Philadelphia, PA: Saunders Elsevier.

Calvey, N. and Williams, N. (2008) *Principles and Practice of Pharmacology for Anaesthetists*. Oxford: Blackwell.

Clayton, B.D. (2009) *Basic Pharmacology for Nurses*, 15th edn. St Louis, MO: Mosby Elsevier.

Coben, D. and Atere-Roberts, E. (2005) *Calculations for Nursing and Healthcare*, 2nd edn. Basingstoke: Palgrave Macmillan.

Downie, G., Mackenzie, J. and Williams, A. (2007) *Pharmacology and Medicines Management for Nurses*, 4th edn. Edinburgh: Churchill Livingstone.

Frisch, A.M., Johnson, A., Timmons, S. and Weatherford, C., (2010) Nurse practitioner role in preparing families for paediatric outpatient surgery, *Paediatric Nursing*, 36(1): 41–6.

Gatford, J.D. and Phillips, N. (2006) *Nursing Calculations*, 7th edn. Edinburgh: Churchill Livingstone Elsevier.

Greenstein, B. (2009) *Clinical Pharmacology for Nurses*, 18th edn. Edinburgh: Churchill Livingstone.

Hutton, M. (2009) *Essential Calculation Skills for Nurses, Midwives and Healthcare Practitioners*. Maidenhead: Open University Press.

Karch, A.M. (2008) *Focus on Nursing Pharmacology*, 4th edn. Philadelphia, PA: Lippincott Williams & Wilkins.

Lapham, R. and Agar, H. (2009) *Drug Calculations for Nurses: A Step-by-step Approach*, 3rd edn. London: Arnold.

Nagelhout, J.J. and Plaus, K.L. (2010) *Handbook of Nurse Anaesthesia*, 4th edn. St Louis, MO: Saunders Elsevier.

Nathanson, M. and Mahahan, R. (2006) *Anaesthesia*. London: Churchill Livingstone.

Peck, T., Hill, S. and Williams, M. (2008) *Pharmacology for Anaesthesia and Critical Care*, 3rd edn. Cambridge: Cambridge University Press.

Pinnock, C., Lin, T. and Smith, T. (2006) *Fundamentals of Anaesthesia*, 2nd edn. Cambridge: Cambridge University Press

Shields, L. and Werder, H. (2002) *Perioperative Nursing*. London: Greenwhich Medical Media.

Simonson, T., Aarbakke, J., Kay, I., Coleman, I., Sinnott, P. and Lyssa, R. (2006) *Illustrated Pharmacology for Nurses*. London: Hodder Arnold.

Starkings, S. and Krause, L. (2010) *Passing Calculation Tests for Nursing Students*. Exeter: Learning Matters.

Wong, A. and Townley, S. (2011) Herbal medicines and anaesthesia, *Continuing Education in Anaesthesia, Critical Care and Pain*, 11(1): 14–17.

6

Vaccines

Learning objectives

After studying this chapter you should be able to:

- Understand the layered defence system of the body which protects against invading micro-organisms.
- Describe the different types of immunity that the body produces.
- Describe the different routes of vaccine administration.
- Understand some of the contraindications to vaccination in specific patient groups.
- Demonstrate a basic understanding of the duration of vaccination protection.

Introduction

The human body is constantly being bombarded by and exposed to infectious agents from the moment of birth. Ideally each person is born with a complete and intact immune system that enables them to resist different kinds of infective and potentially dangerous agents.

Specific and non-specific immunity

The immune system protects the individual from infection using a layered defence of increasing specificity. It has two major subdivisions: the *innate* or *non-specific* immune system and the *adaptive* or *specific* immune system. Non-specific immunity includes physical barriers such as the skin and mucous membranes, and gastric acid and digestive enzymes. Adaptive or specific immunity involves mechanisms that recognize a specific threatening pathogen, or antigen, and produce a specific response to it (it must be learned or may be acquired). If the invader is a bacterial or viral infection there is a time-lag between exposure and maximal response by the body. Specific immunity possesses *memory* – a function of the circulating lymphocytes – which either mediates the specific immune response that is required or divides cells that differentiate into *immune-responsive mediating cells*. Each time the body is exposed to subsequent antigens it serves to strengthen the immune response further.

It is important to remember that both innate and adaptive immunity depend upon the ability of the immune system to distinguish between 'self' and 'non-self' molecules. The body must recognize its 'self-molecules' and 'non-self molecules' because if it attacked *all* molecules it would be destroying the very matrix of its own genetic make-up.

At birth a baby leaves the sterile environment of the womb and is born into a potentially dangerous world of infective micro-organisms and bacteria. In the early hours and days after birth the mother produces a fluid secreted by the mammary glands called *colostrum*. Colostrum is low in fat, and high in carbohydrates, protein and antibodies, in particular *secretory immunoglobulin A* (IgA). If breastfed this will help to protect the baby. Before birth the baby is protected by another antibody, *immunoglobulin G* (IgG) which works through the placenta on the circulatory system. After birth, IgA protects the baby's mucous membranes in the throat, lungs and intestines. Colostrum seals the holes in the gastrointestinal (GI) tract by coating it with a barrier which prevents foreign substances from penetrating. Colostrum also contains high concentrations of leukocytes which aid in the destruction of disease-causing bacteria and viruses; it is also a laxative which helps to clean out meconium (dark greenish/black tarry stool) which in turn decreases the likelihood of jaundice in the infant. Colostrum lasts for about 10–14 days, after which, when the mother's milk has matured, antibodies are still passed but not in the quantities that the colostrum provided. By this process the baby is made naturally immune against many, or all, of the diseases that the mother is immune to. As the immune system matures, the person's own ability to recognize and fight infection becomes a priority.

Once the body has its own antibodies against certain pathogens, antigens and bacteria, this is known as *humoral immunity*.

Humoral immunity

Humoral immunity is an aspect of specific immunity which depends upon the ability of B lymphocytes to recognize specific antigens and initiate a response that protects the body against foreign invasion. The job of the antibodies is to inactivate any antigens and ultimately cause the destruction of any infectious organism. The B cells which mediate humoral immunity do so by producing a single kind of antibody which is displayed on the surface of the B cell itself. Next the antigen binds to one of the surface B cells and the B cell induces those cells either to start producing antibodies or to differentiate into cells that can produce antibodies. B cell differentiation is via 'plasma cells' which are B cells that can immediately produce or secrete antibody molecules, or 'memory cells' which are more stable, long-term B cells that can differentiate into plasma cells.

Active immunity

Active immunization is the induction of immunity by giving an antigen as a vaccine. Antibodies are created by the recipient of the vaccine and may be stored permanently.

Patient group direction

The majority of clinical care is provided on an individual, patient-specific basis. However, in *patient group direction* (PGD) there are specific written instructions for the supply or administration of a licensed named medicine, including vaccines, to specific *groups* of patients who may not be individually identified before presenting for treatment. An example of this is the influenza (flu) vaccination offered at workplaces or by the general practitioner (GP).

Only qualified health professionals may supply or administer medicines under a PGD. This group includes nurses, midwives, health visitors, optometrists, pharmacists, chiropodists, radiographers, orthoptists, physiotherapists and ambulance paramedics. They can only do this as a named individual. It is imperative that health care students never administer, even under the supervision of a mentor, any vaccinations of any description under a PGD. Further information can be found at www.doh.gov.uk/coinh.htm.

Patient-specific direction

A patient-specific direction (PSD) is a written instruction from an independent prescriber such as a doctor, dentist or nurse prescriber to another health care professional. The PSD is given to supply or administer a medicine directly to a named patient or to several named patients.

Types of vaccine

Live attenuated vaccine

This type of vaccine contains a version of the living microbe that has been weakened in a laboratory so that it is unable to cause disease. As it has a weakened form of the disease it is the closest thing to a natural infection. The aim of this type of vaccine is to elicit strong cellular and antibody responses which teach the immune system to respond. Because of this it is possible to provide lifelong immunity with one or two doses. The disadvantages are that the organisms used in attenuated vaccines can change or mutate and there is therefore a possibility that the microbe in the vaccine could revert to a virulent form and cause disease.

Live vaccines are available for measles, mumps and chickenpox and need to be kept refrigerated.

Clinical tip

People who have a damaged or a weakened immune system (e.g. due to chemotherapy or HIV) cannot be given a live vaccine.

Inactivated vaccine

This type of vaccine is produced by killing the disease-causing microbe with heat, radiation or chemicals. Inactivated vaccines are considered to be more stable and safer than live vaccines because the dead microbes cannot mutate back to their disease-causing state. Inactivated vaccines are usually freeze-dried which makes them more accessible to people in developing countries because they do not require refrigeration. The disadvantage is that this type of vaccine stimulates a much weaker immune system response. Therefore it is necessary to administer several additional doses or 'booster' injections to protect a person's immunity. This can be problematic for those without access to regular health care.

Routes of administration

Most vaccines should be given by intramuscular (IM) injection rather than subcutaneously because this method is less likely to cause a local reaction. Oral medication is also a way of delivering a vaccine – for example polio, typhoid and cholera vaccines.

In some developing countries infectious diseases kill an alarming proportion of the child population, making a robust immunization programme highly desirable. However, a proportion of this death rate is owing to the use of non-sterile needles and syringes in the vaccination process itself. As a result, safer methods of vaccination are being developed such as needle-free devices that administer a liquid vaccine through the skin via a high-pressure air jet, or the injection of a 'biosphere' – a tiny starch ball – into the skin. This would have the great advantage of slow release of the vaccine over several months, reducing the need for booster injections.

Because 90 per cent of pathogens gain access via a mucosal route (rectal, vaginal, conjunctival, oral and nasal), vaccines that stimulate the mucosal immune response are highly desirable and as noted above oral vaccines for polio, typhoid and cholera already exist. However, the other mucosal routes, although highly efficient, carry some risk of the development of inflammation and purulent infection.

Administration site

The age of the patient will influence the site of injection. The Royal College of Nursing (RCN) (2000) recommends that infants under the age of 1 should receive all vaccines in the anterolateral aspect of the thigh, because the deltoid muscle of the upper arm, in this age group, is not sufficiently developed. There is also evidence that injecting a vaccine into the gluteal muscle of the buttock of an infant can cause damage to the sciatic nerve. Children who have not yet learned to walk also have a greater level of adipose tissue in that area, which can reduce the absorption and efficacy of the vaccine. For children over the age of 1 the choice of administration site widens, and for older children and adults the deltoid muscle is the preferred site, because it is more developed and far easier to access.

To reduce any adverse effects of vaccination it is important to have a working knowledge of where and when a vaccine may be administered. For example, if more than one vaccine needs to be injected at the same time, they should be given on contralateral (either side) thighs or deltoids depending on the age of the patient. Live-virus vaccines must be given simultaneously and on different sites so that the antibody response is not impaired in any way and the risk of any adverse response is minimized.

How vaccines work

Vaccines work by stimulating the immune system to produce antibodies (immunoglobulin) without the patient actually becoming infected with the particular disease.

Vaccines are designed to trigger the immune system to produce its own antibodies against disease because the direct action of the antibodies makes the body think it has been infected with the disease itself.

> **Clinical tip**
>
> Lymphocytes play an integral role in immunity and are subdivided into B-cell and T-cell types, responsible for humoral and cellular immunity, respectively.

If a person who has been vaccinated comes into contact with the disease itself, their immune system will recognize it and immediately produce the relevant antibodies to fight it. Equally, if a person comes into contact with microbes and has no previous antibodies for defence against them (passive immunity), they become immunized because the immune system will eventually create its own antibodies and other defences. If the person is then exposed to the invading microbe again, the memory of the previous invasion triggers the immune response very quickly. The immune response is very efficient in recognizing and destroying the microbe and the person is said to be immune. Childhood diseases are a good example of this: children only get infected once by certain microbes and are then deemed to be immune from them for life.

> **Clinical tip**
>
> The T in T cell stands for 'thymus' and it is in the thymus that T cells mature, especially in immature immune systems (children). B cells are not matured in the thymus. B lymphocytes are the producers of antibodies.

There will always be some individuals for whom vaccination is contraindicated and should be deferred. It is important to remember that advice should always be sought from a doctor or consultant about withholding a specific vaccine for certain medical conditions and contraindications.

Patients should not be given a vaccination if:

- they have had a confirmed anaphylactic reaction to a previous dose of a vaccine containing the same antigen;

Box 6.1 Contraindications and risk groups

Contraindication	Risk group
Egg allergy	Children with an egg allergy who are due to receive measles, mumps and rubella (MMR) vaccine will normally be able to have the vaccination; however, individuals with a confirmed anaphylactic reaction to eggs should not receive influenza or yellow fever vaccines.
Pregnancy	As there is a theoretical concern that vaccinating a pregnant woman with a live vaccine may infect the foetus, live vaccines are generally delayed until after the birth of the baby.
Immunosuppression	Any patients that are immunosuppressed due to chemotherapy, radiotherapy, bone marrow transplant, HIV, or any combined immunodeficiency syndrome should not receive a live vaccine, as these can cause severe or fatal infections. In these circumstances inactivated vaccines may be administered although they elicit a much lower response in these patients.
HIV infection	Due to the complexities of this disease process and the variety of ages that the condition affects, some vaccines will be contraindicated at certain times. Vaccinations are tailored to meet the requirements of the patient.

- they have a confirmed anaphylactic reaction to another component contained within the vaccine.

Risk groups

Box 6.1 lists some specific contraindications for certain risk groups in society – it is not an exhaustive list.

Immunization in children

Vaccination of children begins from the age of 2 months and can take place up to the age of 18. In the UK all children are routinely offered vaccinations against key diseases as part of the national childhood immunization schedule, which is designed to protect against the diseases listed in Box 6.2.

In 2008 a vaccine against human papilloma virus (HPV) was introduced for 12–13-year-old girls. The vaccine protects against two strains of HPV known to cause cervical cancer. Current studies show that the protection of this vaccination lasts for at least five years, although further studies are ongoing to establish whether a booster will be needed. The vaccine is not available for boys at present, despite evidence showing that HPV has been linked to cancers of the penis, oral cavity and anus. Some strains of HPV also cause genital warts in both males and females.

Bacillus Calmette-Guérin

Tuberculosis (TB) is a bacterial infection which affects the lungs, but may also affect the brain and bones. In most instances the infection remains latent (hidden and not yet developed) and asymptomatic (showing no symptoms); however, when it is active it carries a high mortality rate in developing countries. Bacillus Calmette-Guérin (BCG) is a vaccine against TB that is prepared from the weakened (live) bovine tuberculosis bacillus *Mycobacterium bovis*. The BCG vaccine is about

Box 6.2 Childhood immunization in the UK

Illness	Period of protection
Diphtheria	At least 10 years
Polio	Lifelong protection
Whooping cough	At least 3 years
Tetanus	At least 10 years
Measles	Long-lasting protection
Mumps	Long-lasting protection
Rubella	Long-lasting protection
Hib (Haemophilus influenza type B)	Long-lasting protection
Meningitis C	Long-lasting protection
Pneumococcal (streptococcus) pneumonia	Long-lasting protection

80 per cent effective in preventing tuberculosis for approximately 15 years.

The BCG immunization programme was introduced into the UK in 1953 and the vaccine given to school children around the age of 13 years. The programme ceased in 2005 due to the declining number of TB cases in the UK population. The BCG vaccine is now only recommended for infants and children at high risk of the developing the disease.

Method of administration

Prior to the administration of BCG a skin test called a 'reactive tuberculin test' is conducted. This is designed to reveal any positive tuberculin reaction. If such a reaction is observed the patient will not receive BCG because there is a high risk of severe local inflammation and possible scarring. Such children should be screened for active tuberculosis.

BCG is given as a single intradermal injection at the insertion of the deltoid muscle onto the humerus near the middle of the upper arm. This site is most frequently used because local complications are relatively rare.

Side-effects

A local reaction may be observed in the appearance of a papule (small circumscribed elevation of the skin) at the site of vaccination, usually within two to six weeks. The papule flattens and widens, causing a small amount of scaling and crusting, and eventually develops into a small ulcer. If natural healing is allowed to take place, after six weeks there will be a scar, approximately 4mm in diameter.

Contraindications

The BCG vaccine should not be given to patients:

- who have past history of TB;
- who have a positive pre-immunization tuberculin test;
- who are HIV positive;
- who are pregnant;
- who have had a previous BCG vaccination.

Case studies

① Your mentor asks you to explain how a newborn baby that is being breast fed will develop natural immunity against certain disease processes.

- How will you respond?

② A patient has just received a vaccination. He asks you to explain what the vaccination will do to his immune system once it enters his body.

- How would you explain active immunity to him?

Key learning points

Introduction

➤ Each person is ideally born with a complete and intact immune system.

Specific and non-specific immunity

➤ The immune system protects the individual from infection via a layered defence of increasing specificity.
➤ There are two major subdivisions – the innate or non-specific immune system and the adaptive, specific immune system.

Humoral immunity

➤ Is an aspect of specific immunity which depends on the ability of B lymphocytes to recognize specific antigens and initiate a response to protect the body from foreign invasion.
➤ B lymphocytes differentiate through plasma cells and memory cells.

Active immunity

➤ Active immunity is the induction of immunity by giving an antigen as a vaccine.
➤ Antibodies are created by the recipient of the vaccine and may be stored permanently.

Patient group direction

➤ Only qualified and named health professionals may supply or administer medicine under a PGD.
➤ Students are not allowed to administer a PGD, even under supervision.

Live attenuated vaccines

➤ Contain a version of the living microbe that has been weakened in a laboratory so that it is unable to cause disease.
➤ Can elicit strong cellular and antibody responses within the body which teaches the immune system to respond.

Inactivated vaccines

➤ These vaccines are produced by killing the disease-causing microbe with heat, radiation or chemicals.
➤ Considered to be more stable and safer than live vaccines.

Routes of administration

➤ Most vaccines are given by IM injection rather than subcutaneously.

→

←

Administration site

➢ The age of the patient determines the site of administration.

How vaccines work

➢ Vaccines work by stimulating the immune system to produce antibodies without the person actually becoming infected.

Risk groups

➢ There is a risk to patients who suffer from egg alergy, who are pregnant, who are immuno-suppressed or who are infected with HIV.

Immunization in children

➢ In the UK children are routinely offered vaccinations against key diseases.

Bacillus Calmette-Guérin

➢ A vaccine against TB that is approximately 80 per cent effective in preventing TB for around 15 years.
➢ Prior to the administration of BCG a skin test called a 'reactive tuberculin test' is conducted.
➢ BCG is given as a single intradermal injection at the insertion of the deltoid muscle of the upper arm.
➢ A papule at the site of vaccination may appear, usually within two to six weeks.
➢ BCG should not be given to patients with a past history of TB, following a positive pre-immunization tuberculin test, to those who are HIV positive individuals or to patients who are pregnant.

Multiple choice questions

1 What types of patient should avoid vaccines containing live viruses?

a) Pregnant patients
b) Immunosuppressed patients
c) HIV patients
d) All of the above

2 Patient's should not be given any type of vaccination if

a) They have had a confirmed anaphylactic reaction to a previous dose of vaccine containing the same antigen

→

←

b) They are only youngsters
c) They have an egg allergy
d) They are breast feeding

3 In 2008 a new vaccine was introduced in the UK for 12–13-year-old girls, what was it for?

a) Chlamydia
b) Pelvic inflammatory disease
c) Human papilloma virus (HPV)
d) Syphilis

4 The BCG vaccine should not be given to patients with

a) Eczema
b) Mild illness (no fever)
c) Recent exposure to infectious disease
d) Previous BCG vaccination

5 Active immunity is

a) Antibodies that are passed from mother to foetus
b) A vaccine designed to trigger the immune system to produce its own antibodies against disease
c) A vaccine that suppresses the immune response
d) Protection for the body that is only temporary

6 Live vaccines should be stored in a

a) Dark cupboard
b) Warm oven
c) Refrigerator
d) Sunny place

7 For an infant under the age of 1 the preferred injection site for a vaccine is

a) Anterolateral thigh (high up)
b) Buttocks
c) An area of increased adipose tissue
d) Anterolateral thigh (low down)

8 The three oral vaccines that are already available are

a) MMR
b) Polio, typhoid, cholera
c) Whooping cough, polio, hepatitis A
d) Diptheria, influenza, measles

→

 ←

9 B lymphocytes are the producers of

a) Lymphocytes
b) Interferon
c) Antibodies
d) Lysozymes

10 PGD should be administered by

a) A student nurse/midwife
b) A named, qualified health care professional
c) Health care assistants
d) Medical students

Recommended further reading

Barber, P. and Robertson, D. (2012) *Essentials of Pharmacology for Nurses*, 2nd edn. Maidenhead: Open University Press.

Beckwith, S. and Franklin, P. (2007) *Oxford Handbook of Nurse Prescribing*. Oxford: Oxford University Press.

Brenner, G.M. and Stevens, C.W. (2009) *Pharmacology*, 3rd edn. Philadelphia, PA: Saunders Elsevier.

Clayton, B.D. (2009) *Basic Pharmacology for Nurses*, 15th edn. St Louis, MO: Mosby Elsevier.

Coben, D. and Atere-Roberts, E. (2005) *Calculations for Nursing and Healthcare*, 2nd edn. Basingstoke: Palgrave Macmillan.

Downie, G., Mackenzie, J. and Williams, A. (2007) *Pharmacology and Medicines Management for Nurses*, 4th edn. Edinburgh: Churchill Livingstone.

Gatford, J.D. and Phillips, N. (2006) *Nursing Calculations*, 7th edn. Edinburgh: Churchill Livingstone Elsevier.

Greenstein, B. (2009) *Clinical Pharmacology for Nurses*, 18th edn. Edinburgh: Churchill Livingstone.

Hutton, M. (2009) *Essential Calculation Skills for Nurses, Midwives and Healthcare Practitioners*. Maidenhead: Open University Press.

Karch, A.M. (2008) *Focus on Nursing Pharmacology*, 4th edn. Philadelphia, PA: Lippincott Williams & Wilkins.

Lapham, R. and Agar, H. (2009) *Drug Calculations for Nurses: A Step-by-step Approach*, 3rd edn. London: Arnold.

National Health Service Executive (2000) *Patient Group Directions*. London: Department of Health.

RCN (Royal College of Nursing) (2001) *UK Guidance on Best Practice in Vaccine Administration*. London: RCN.

Simonson, T., Aarbakke, J., Kay, I., Coleman, I., Sinnott, P. and Lyssa, R. (2006) *Illustrated Pharmacology for Nurses*. London: Hodder Arnold.

Starkings, S. and Krause, L. (2010) *Passing Calculation Tests for Nursing Students*. Exeter: Learning Matters.

Intravenous fluids and nutrition

7

Chapter contents

Learning objectives

After studying this chapter you should be able to:

- Understand your responsibilities when delivering a drug or fluid infusion to a patient.
- Demonstrate a basic understanding of the different veins and routes used in the delivery of intravenous infusions.
- Describe fluid and electrolyte imbalance and the measures needed to correct them.
- Share an understanding of the complications that may arise with delivery of intravenous fluid/nutrition and the measures taken to avoid them.
- Use basic maths to calculate simple drug dosages in relation to fluids and nutrition.

Introduction

One of the most important aspects of a nurse's job is the administration of a prescribed medication. This may take the form of oral tablets, intravenous (IV) medication/solutions, injections and enteral nutrition. The Nursing and Midwifery Council's (NMC) (2007) *Standards for Medicine Management* clearly sets out the requirements of a registrant (qualified nurse) and the bounds of their professional accountability. This chapter aims to introduce you to some of the advantages and disadvantages of IV administration and the professional accountability to be exercised in terms of the best interests of the patient. In brief, the NMC (2007: 7) sets out the following standards and guidelines.

- You must be certain of the identity of the patient to whom the medicine is to be administered.
- You must check that the patient is not allergic to the medicine before administering it.
- You must know the therapeutic uses of the medicine: its normal dosage, side-effects, precautions and contraindications.
- You must be aware of the patient's plan of care (care plan or pathway).
- You must check that the prescription or the label on the medicine is clearly written and unambiguous.
- You must check the expiry date (where it exists) of the medicine to be administered.
- You must have considered the dosage, weight (where appropriate), method of administration, route and timing.
- You must administer or withhold in the context of the patient's condition (e.g. digoxin is not usually to be given if the pulse is below 60) and coexisting therapies, such as physiotherapy.
- You must contact the prescriber or another authorized person without delay where contraindications are discovered, where the patient develops a reaction to the medicine, or where assessment of the patient indicates that the medicine is no longer suitable.

Nurses and midwives are accountable for their practice and must always be able to justify the decisions they make. The law states that if a patient's needs exceed the health care professional's skills or abilities, then he or she should bring this to the attention of the senior nurse in charge and not attempt to meet the patient's needs unsupported.

Where medication, in any of its guises, is involved, a health care professional remains accountable for monitoring and evaluating the effectiveness of the prescribed therapy and ensuring that relevant documentation reflects the patient's response, any adverse effects and any therapeutic benefits. The administration of any medication or solution should, at all times, be accompanied by a signed prescription from a doctor or authorized nurse prescriber. Clear documentation should indicate whether the medication was administered, withheld or declined.

Anatomy and physiology

Most blood vessels have a similar construction (with the exception of the capillaries). The walls of all blood vessels, arteries and veins are composed of three layers of tissue called *tunica*.

Tunica externa

The outer layer, *tunica externa* (adventitia) is composed of connective tissue, collagen and nerve fibres. It surrounds and supports the vessel with sympathetic nerve fibres that transmit nerve impulses to keep the walls of the vessel in a state of *tonus* which stops the vessel from collapsing in on itself. The infiltration of sympathetic nerve fibres can constrict the walls of the vessel when impulses are increased (vasoconstriction) and allow for dilation of the vessel walls when nerve impulses are decreased (vasodilation). Generally there is more fibrous tissue found in arteries than in veins.

Tunica media

The middle layer is called the *tunica media* and is made up of vascular smooth muscle supported by a layer of collagen and elastin fibres. The smooth muscle cells that make up this layer produce the vasoconstriction/dilation of the blood vessel by releasing the neurotransmitter norepinephrine which diffuses into the tunica media and acts upon the nearby smooth muscle cells.

Tunica intima

The inner layer is known as the *tunica intima* and consists of a single layer of flattened endothelial cells with little subendothelial connective tissue. Beneath the tissue is an internal elastic lamina (thin layer) that is well developed in muscular arteries. Endothelial cells form a continuous lining throughout the vascular system called the *endothelium*. The endothelium plays a role in vascular resistance, control of platelet adhesion and clotting. Capillaries are only composed of endothelial cells with few or no elastic fibres; this aids the rapid exchange of water and solutes between the tissue fluid and blood plasma. Endothelial cells can be easily damaged as a result of the rapid advancement of a cannula or siting a cannula that is too large for the lumen of the vein. Another cause of endothelial damage is the rapid infusion of large quantities of fluid that the vessel may find difficult to accommodate.

Veins used in intravenous therapy

The most commonly used veins for peripheral and central venous therapy are:

- Internal jugular
- External jugular
- Superior vena cava
- Left subclavian
- Cephalic – large vein for venipuncture
- Basilic – straight, strong vein for venipuncture
- Median cubital
- Median cephalic
- Median antebrachial – a last resort when no other means are available
- Accessory cephalic – readily accepts large-gauge needles
- Dorsal venous arch
- Metacarpal – easily accessible, less likely to dislodge
- Digital – may be used for short-term therapy

Fluid

Fluid compartments

Body fluids are mainly composed of water with certain substances dissolved within this. The average adult body contains between 40–45 litres of water, which equates to about two-thirds of total body weight. The abundance of water within the body needs a balanced approach to provide the optimum environment for the tissues and organs to survive. About 25 litres of water is selectively stored within cells (intracellular). Of this, 3 litres of water is found within blood cells (blood is approximately 91 per cent water), and extracellular fluid (fluid that surrounds the cells) makes up the remaining amount. This can be further broken down into *interstitial fluid* (12 litres), blood plasma (3 litres) and transcellular fluids (1–3 litres). Transcellular fluids include cerebrospinal fluid around the brain and spinal cord. To maintain a balance, fluids that are distributed between the intracellular and extracellular compartments must remain constant.

For a female the amount of water within the body is approximately 50 per cent, and for a male 60 per cent. This is because men generally have less body fat and more lean muscle than women, although there are always exceptions. It follows that the percentage of water in a patient who is very emaciated (excessive leanness) will be much higher than for an obese patient.

Throughout a person's lifespan there are a number of issues to consider regarding water percentages and body fat. In infancy there is a greater storage of body water in the interstitial spaces than in adults, with about 15 per cent typically being made up of interstitial fluid. This balances out in adulthood as more lean muscle is developed. As a person ages beyond 60 years and skeletal muscle mass declines, the proportion of fat within the body increases and water content drops to about 45 per cent.

The average healthy adult consumes about 2–2.5 litres of water a day from food and drink, and the oxidation of food during metabolism produces between 200–300ml per day. A healthy individual has an equivalent fluid *loss* of 2–2.4 litres per day. This maintains *homeostasis*.

In illness a patient's consumption of food and fluids may be altered and their fluid input/output may be severely compromised, ultimately leading to dehydration which can affect fluid and electrolyte balance. This may necessitate the administration of fluids by IV infusion.

Fluid types

Isotonic fluid is made up of normal saline (0.9 per cent) and glucose (5 per cent) in water. It is a solution that has the same solute concentration (or *osmolarity*) as that within the body. Infusing the solution doesn't alter the concentration of serum and therefore osmosis does not occur. As a result the isotonic solution remains where it is infused (inside the blood vessel), which does not affect the size of the cell.

Hypotonic fluid is made up of saline (0.45 per cent) ('half-normal' saline), and dextrose (2.5 per cent) in water. It is a fluid with a lower osmotic pressure relative to another fluid. It has a lower solute concentration than serum. As a result fluid shifts out of the blood vessels and into the cells and interstitial spaces, where the solute concentration is higher.

Hypertonic fluid (10 per cent dextrose), as can be found in what is known as total parenteral nutrition (TPN) is a fluid with a higher osmotic pressure relative to another fluid. As a result, infusing a hypertonic solution increases the solute concentration of serum. This pulls fluid from the cells and interstitial fluid by osmosis.

Fluid balance

Fluid balance in a healthy person is managed automatically. A person's daily intake is approximately 2600ml, usually made up of liquids (1500ml) and solid food (800ml), along with water produced from oxidation (300ml). Daily output (loss) is also approximately 2600ml, made up of output via the skin (600ml), lungs (400ml) and kidneys (1500ml), and as faeces (100ml).

Fluid loss is divided into *sensible* and *insensible* loss. Sensible fluid loss occurs through urination, faeces, vomit and wound exudates and is so called because the fluid loss is measurable and observable. Insensible fluid loss occurs through the skin (sweating – this can be greatly affected by humidity) and lungs (breathing – this can be affected by respiratory depth and rate). If the fluid loss is excessive (perhaps due to diarrhoea and sickness) then the body runs the risk of dehydration. This is detected by *osmoreceptors* found in the hypothalamus of the brain. These modified nerve cells then release an anti-diuretic hormone (vasopressin) which reduces the volume of urine leaving the kidneys by promoting the rapid uptake of water by osmosis (under the influence of osmotic pressure) into the renal medulla.

Electrolytes

Electrolytes are a major component of body fluids and there are seven major types (see Box 7.1). Electrolytes can be either *extracellular* (outside the cell membrane) or *intracellular* (inside the cell membrane).

Fluid and electrolyte imbalances

If a person is adequately taking in the correct amount of food and fluid per day then homeostasis should be maintained. The body relies upon its daily input/output to do this but may become compromised by a decrease in circulating fluid volume. This can become an emergency situation, in some instances, very quickly. Box 7.2 outlines some of the conditions that may necessitate fluid replacement therapy.

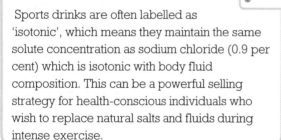

Clinical tip

Sports drinks are often labelled as 'isotonic', which means they maintain the same solute concentration as sodium chloride (0.9 per cent) which is isotonic with body fluid composition. This can be a powerful selling strategy for health-conscious individuals who wish to replace natural salts and fluids during intense exercise.

Box 7.1 The major electrolytes

Extracellular electrolytes		Normal levels
Sodium	Aids nerve and muscle fibre impulse transmission	135–145mEq/L (Sl, 135–145mmol/L)
Chloride	Maintains serum osmolarity (along with sodium)	100–108mEq/L (Sl, 100–108mmol/L)
Calcium – ionized	Helps maintain cell membrane structure, function and permeability	4.65–5.2mg/dl (Sl, 1.1–1.25mmol/L)
Intracellular electrolytes		
Potassium	Responsible for cell excitability, nerve impulse conduction, myocardial membrane responsiveness	3.5–5mEq/L (Sl, 3.5–5mmol/L)
Phosphorous	Responsible for energy metabolism. Plays an essential role in muscle, red blood cell and neurological function	2.7–4.5mg/dl (Sl, 0.87–1.45mmol/L)
Magnesium	Facilitates Na+ and K+ movement across all membranes	1.3–2.1mEq/L (Sl, 1.3–2.1mmol/L)
Bicarbonate	Present in extracellular fluid. Primary function is regulating acid-base balance	22–28mEq/L (SI, 22–28mmol/L)

Intravenous infusion

IV thereapy or infusion is commonly called a 'drip' because the method of delivery employs a drip chamber which prevents air entering the body. This type of therapy is the fastest way to deliver fluid, transfuse blood, correct electrolyte imbalances, alleviate dehydration and administer medications throughout the body.

Therapy is administered via a *peripheral vein*, which is any vein that is not in the chest or abdomen. Hand and arm veins are traditionally used although it is possible to use veins in the feet and legs. Veins are prefered over arteries because the flow of fluid will pass through the lungs *first*, before passing through the body.

Peripheral cannulas are the most common IV access method. A peripheral cannula consists of a short catheter that is introduced through the skin into a peripheral vein. It is made of a flexible plastic mounted on a metal *trocar* (introducing needle).

Once the tip of the needle and cannula are located in a suitable vein the trocar is withdrawn and then disposed of in accordance with sharps policy. The cannula is advanced inside the vein to an appropriate position and then secured using a suitable dressing. The reason blood may be removed on the introduction of the newly sited cannula is that the cannula fills up with blood on insertion, whether a blood sample is taken or not. However, on subsequent occasions blood would be drawn back into the catheter and a volume of blood would be left in the catheter after the sample had been withdrawn. As this blood is flushed back into the vein as the cannula was cleared with injectable saline, infection from the catheter port may also be flushed into the bloodstream. This then has the potential to greatly increase the risk of an infection passing back to the patient.

A peripheral cannula cannot be left in the vein indefinitely because of the risk of *phlebitis*

Box 7.2 Conditions that may require fluid replacement therapy

Dehydration	Quite common in elderly patients. If it becomes severe it may lead to the reduction in the circulating volume and *hypovolaemia* (reduced volume of blood in the circulation)
Increase in temperature	This leads to vasodilation (widening of the lumen of the blood vessel) which can increase fluid space, resulting in symptoms of reduced circulating blood volume
Loss of whole blood	The most common reason for the loss of circulating blood volume. May result from surgery or personal injury
Loss of plasma	This can occur if a person receives partial-thickness or full-thickness burns that occupy more than 20 per cent of the total body surface
Bleeding disorders	May result from any type of platelet (cells that encourage clotting) or coagulation disease/disorder, including *thrombocytopenia* (reduction of the number of platelets) or *thrombocytosis* (increase in the number of platelets). Either of these conditions can cause or fail to prevent internal or external bleeding

(inflammation of a vein), *cellulitis* (inflammation of the skin and connective tissue) and *bacteraemia* (the presence of bacteria in the blood).

Clinical tip

Hospital policy usually dictates that IV sites are relocated every two to three days and that unused IV access is removed after 24 hours.

If peripheral IV access is not attainable, central IV lines can be considered in certain patients. Central lines deliver fluids and medications via a catheter that has its tip within a large vein, usually the superior or inferior vena cava, or within the right atrium of the heart. The advantages of using a central line are that it can deliver fluids and medication which will reach the heart immediately and will be distributed to the rest of the body very quickly. As central lines can have multiple ports (three lines into one general line), multiple medications can be delivered at the same time. A further advantage is that medical staff can measure cen-

tral venous pressure through the line. Despite the obvious advantages, central lines are not without risk and in some instances can carry a higher risk of bleeding, bacteraemia and air embolism.

Risks

Any breach or break in the skin's integrity carries a risk of infection. Although IV access is performed as a sterile procedure, skin-colonization of *Staph. auras* or *Candida albicans* may enter the body via the introducing needle. Infection at IV sites usually remains local and there may be visible swelling, redness and pain which can be accompanied by fever. If bacteria do get into the bloodstream the infection is likely to be septicaemia which can have life-threatening consequences. Central lines ultimately pose a greater risk of septicaemia as the line delivers the bacteria directly into the central circulation.

When a cannula or central line is sited it is not necessary to shave any hair away with a razor. Shaving with a razor can cause *microabrasions* (small cuts in the skin) which potentially increase the risk of infection. The same applies to any *depilatories* (creams used to remove hair) as there is a risk of allergic reaction or irritation to the skin.

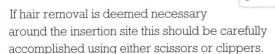

Clinical tip

If hair removal is deemed necessary around the insertion site this should be carefully accomplished using either scissors or clippers.

The skin should be rubbed for approximately 30 seconds with an antimicrobial solution to decontaminate the area effectively. The skin should then be allowed to air-dry for approximately 30 seconds before proceeding with the vascular access device. For peripheral cannulae a 2 per cent chlorhexidine in alcohol solution should be applied to the site for 30 seconds.

Once IV access is gained each device should be stabilized in a manner that does not interfere with the assessment and monitoring of the IV site, or impede the delivery of the prescribed therapy. Types of stabilizing product include transparent semipermeable membrane (TSM) dressing, sterile tape, sutures and surgical strips. Dressings whose integrity has become compromised must be replaced immediately.

Nurses have a duty to monitor insertion sites by visual inspection and palpation for tenderness on a daily basis to check for potential risks or infections. Most hospital trusts endorse visual infusion phlebitis charts to assist health care staff in taking the approriate action. Local policy guidelines should always be followed, and the insertion site should be observed and documented at least once per shift.

Clinical tip

Documentation in the nursing notes should reflect routine assessment of the site(s) and describe their condition on a regular basis.

Phlebitis

Phlebitis is an inflammation of a vein that can be caused by infection, the presence of the cannula, IV medication or fluid that is being infused through it. It can often be caused by using a vein that is too small for the IV therapy or a vascular access device that is too large for the vein. A complication that may further arise is the development of *thrombophlebitis* which is an irritation of the vein resulting in the formation of a clot and is usually more painful than the phlebitis itself. If a clot is dislodged and enters the pulmonary system it can lead to a pulmonary embolus (PE).

Phlebitis can follow any infusion or the simple injection of a single drug. It is however more common after a continuous infusion. Distal veins (those furthest from the heart) are particularly susceptible. Most single injections don't usually cause phlebitis when administered correctly; however, phenytoin (epilepsy medication) and diazepam (anxiolytic) can produce phlebitis after one or more injections at the same IV site.

Clinical tip

Symptoms of phlebitis can often mimic those of infection: warmth, swelling, pain, increased temperature and redness around the site of insertion. In all cases the IV line should be removed and the patient's vital signs carefully observed.

Infiltration

This happens when the tip of the IV cannula withdraws from the vein or protrudes through the vein into the surrounding tissue, allowing fluid or blood to seep in: the cannula is said to have 'tissued'. The cannula must be removed and re-sited at a different location. Failure to do this may lead to a compression injury (nerve damage due to the build-up of surrounding fluid pressing upon the nerve; if not relieved this can lead to permanent damage). Infiltration commonly occurs when an IV cannula has been improperly placed or has become dislodged.

In elderly patients this type of complication may occur because their veins are much thinner and more fragile.

The complications of infiltration include:

- Slow flow rate
- Blanching (becoming white or pale)
- Swelling
- Discomfort
- Tightness

Clinical tip

If any of these complications arise the infusion should be stopped and re-sited. The offended insertion site should be elevated and can have warm soaks applied to it.

The risk of infiltration increases when the IV access device remains in the vein for more than two days or when the tip of the cannula is positioned near a flexion area (e.g. elbow or wrist) because the normal movement of such joints may cause the device to dislodge or damage the lumen of the vessel.

Fluid overload

This occurs when IV fluids are given at a higher rate or in a larger volume than the system can absorb or excrete. Possible signs and symptoms of circulatory overload include respiratory distress, elevated blood pressure, positive fluid balance and neck vein distension or engorgement. Elderly patients and those with cardiac problems are particularly vulnerable to developing fluid overload.

Administration of too-dilute or too-concentrated a solution can also disrupt a patient's electrolyte balance. Therefore, regular blood tests should be carried out to monitor electrolyte parameters.

Speed shock

Speed shock is a reaction that occurs when a substance is rapidly introduced to the circulatory sys-

tem. It can occur when any IV solutions/drugs are given or infused too rapidly, including bolus injections. The patient will almost immediately suffer facial flushing, an irregular pulse, headache and hypotension (low blood pressure). Loss of consciousness and cardiac arrest may also occur.

Clinical tip

If speed shock occurs during IV administration, clamp the IV set immediately, notify the person in charge, provide oxygen and monitor the patient's vital signs.

Air embolism

Just how much air within the circulatory system a person can tolerate varies from patient to patient. Small amounts of air entering an IV system can usually be filtered out by the pulmonary circulation. However, more than 5ml/kg of air displaced into the IV space can cause significant injury. Critically ill patients are unable to tolerate large amounts of air and fatalities have been reported in this patient group with as little as 10ml of air.

If very small amounts of air do enter the venous system they are broken up in the capillary bed and absorbed from the circulation without producing any symptoms. There have been reports, however, that complications have arisen from as little as 20ml of air (the length of an unprimed IV giving set) injected intravenously. This reiterates the importance of ensuring that the line is primed correctly with the correct fluid in accordance with the manufacturer's instructions.

The closer a vein is to the right side of the heart the lower the amount of air that is needed to prove fatal: 0.5ml of air in the left anterior descending artery can cause ventricular fibrillation leading to cardiac arrest and possible death. With a venous air embolism it is quite common for resultant tachyarrhythmias (fast heart rate and rhythms) and bradyarrhythmias (slower heart rate and rhythms) to occur.

An air embolism is less likely to occur with a peripheral cannula but the risk increases with a central line.

When an air embolism enters the right side of the heart (right atrium) it puts a substantial strain on the right ventricle which can also cause a rise in pulmonary artery pressure. This increase can lead to right ventricular outflow obstruction which will further compromise pulmonary venous return to the left atrium/ventricle. This diminished pulmonary venous return ultimately leads to decreased ventricular preload which culminates in a decreased cardiac output and eventually to the collapse of the systemic system. In simple terms this means that the amount of air entering the right side of the heart compromises the blood flow forward via the pulmonary artery, which takes deoxygenated blood back to the lungs. Therefore, insufficient oxygenated blood returns to the left side of the heart via the pulmonary veins. The air embolism has interrupted the normal preload (the stretching of the muscle fibres in the ventricles resulting from blood volume) which also affects contractility (influenced by preload – the greater the stretch the more forceful the contraction) and afterload (the pressure that the ventricular muscles must generate to overcome the higher pressure of the aorta to get the blood out of the heart). The result is that the heart no longer beats rhythmically, increasing the risk of the patient developing cardiac arrhythmias.

Preparation and procedure

Wherever possible an IV medication is checked with two registrants, or in exceptional circumstances the registrant and another competent person, prior to its administration.

Prior to administration the nurse should appropriately label any containers, vials and syringes correctly, identify the correct patient and ensure all checks for allergies, content, dose, rate, route and any expiry date are thoroughly adhered too. All

Box 7.3 Air embolism

Signs of air embolism
1 Loss of consciousness/collapse
2 Acute respiratory distress
3 Hypotension
4 Weak pulse/reduced cardiac output
5 Increased jugular venous pressure
6 Chest pain

Immediate treatment
1 Seek emergency help
2 Locate source and prevent further entrainment (e.g. clamp IV tubing),close open stopcocks, ports or three-way taps
3 Lay the patient flat
4 Tip the bed head down and turn patient onto their left side with their head lower than their feet (modified Trendelenburg position). This will decrease the flow of air into the vein during inspiration by decreasing intrathoracic pressure. The air bubble will then rise into the right ventricle, relieving the obstruction to the pulmonary vasculature bed
5 Administer 100 per cent oxygen via a face mask, *not* a nasal cannula
6 Monitor observations
7 Stay with the patient and offer reassurance
8 Document incident

Complications
1 Shock
2 Death
3 Neurological injury
4 Myocardial infarction

medications to be administered must have been signed by an appropriate doctor or nurse pre-scriber. This done, the following procedure should be followed.

- Ensure all infusion systems are checked for any signs of damage or defects.
- Check infusion bag for expiry date.
- Close all the clamps of the giving set. Pierce the infusion with the spike of the giving set and gently squeeze the drip chamber until it is half filled with fluid. Once half filled, open all clamps of the giving set, allowing free flow of the IV fluid to fully prime the line.
- If any air bubbles in the line are visible, purge the line further until all evidence of air bubbles is eradicated.
- Ensure that before the line is attached to the patient via a Luer-lock, there is no air in the line evident and the drip chamber remains half filled.
- Make sure the line is connected correctly and securely to the correct patient having checked their prescription sheet.
- Ensure the fluid is run through at the correct speed (if a pump is used) or the correct amount of drips per minute if no pump is required.

During the infusion:

- Observe the line regularly for any air bubbles.
- Observe the administered fluid regularly to ensure it has not run out.
- Check the IV tubing does not run dry. If this happens the tubing will need either to be re-placed, ensuring the new line is purged to erad-icate any air bubbles, or to be detached from the patient and purged of any air before recon-necting the bag and returning the line to the patient. If the line becomes detached ensure it is closed off with a bung to prevent any air en-tering the venous system.
- Always ensure that the roller clamps are closed when fluid bags are changed.

Clinical tip

Air bubbles that are very tiny (pin-head bubbles) can be left, as long as they are not excessive, but should be monitored if air in the line is detected. In the case of excessive air bubbles, stop the infusion and clamp the line shut using the roller clamp. Then follow the above advice for the eradication of air in the line.

Infusion systems

There are a number of specific types of infusion system that are designed to deliver a measured amount of drugs or fluids by either IV or subcu-taneous (SC) routes. Their aim is to specifically de-liver a set amount over a specific period of time to within a desired therapeutic range.

Gravity flow infusions

Gravity infusion devices depend entirely on gravity to drive the infusion. The administration set has a drip chamber and a roller clamp (which controls the flow of the fluid/drug) which is usually mea-sured by counting the number of drops per minute. Gravity flow infusion devices are often used when there is no precedent to deliver a precise regimen of a fluid/drug in an exact amount of time to a pa-tient whose medical condition gives no cause for concern or anticipated complications.

The flow rate is based on the volume to be in-fused, the number of hours that the infusion will run and the drop rate of the administration set.

The equation is:

$$\frac{\text{Volume to be infused} \times \text{Drop rate}}{\text{Time (e.g. 60 minutes)}}$$

$$= \text{Drops per minute}$$

It is important to consider the drops per minute that the administration set recommends. For a crystal-loid (e.g. normal saline) it is 20 drops/ml); for a blood administration set it is 15 drops/ml.

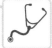

Clinical tip

Always check the IV administration set to calculate the volume in drops. You need to know how many drops of fluid ordered are contained in 1ml. You should find this information on the packaging of the administration set. The volume in ml is then multiplied by the number of drops per ml to give the volume in drops. Similarly, to find the rate in minutes, you need to change the hours into minutes by multiplying by 60.

This type of system is easy to set up, generally familiar to members of staff and low cost. However, the rate of infusion can be affected by the condition and size of the vein used to deliver the fluid, the viscosity (stickiness) of the fluid, the temperature of the fluid and the height of the container (any changes in height will alter the flow rate). The disadvantages include a risk of 'free flow' (the fluid enters the body unimpeded). There can be a variation in the droplet size infused and this requires frequent observations and adjustments by medical staff.

Volumetric pumps
Volumetric pumps work using a linear peristaltic pumping mechanism (a wave-like pushing of fluid out of a chamber). They calculate the volume of fluid to be administered and measure the volume displaced in a reservoir which is an integral component of the giving set. These pumps are designed to overcome resistance to flow with an increased delivery pressure and therefore do not rely on gravity to deliver the fluid. They are able to deliver crystalloid and colloid fluids as well as blood products and have a wide range of features, including air-in-line detectors and comprehensive alarm systems. However, they are relatively expensive and often require a dedicated administration set. Using the wrong type of administration set for the pump can result in a drug/fluid error even if the pump appears to be working.

Volumetric pumps have the facility to work with either mains electricity or a battery. It is best prac-

tice to plug the pump into a mains socket by the bedside if the patient is not ambulatory (mobile). Volumetric pumps should always be plugged into the mains to preserve the battery life when not in use. The cadmium batteries usually last for approximately two to three hours, allowing the patient to continue to receive medication via this method even if they leave the bedside. The pumps are programmed to between 1 and 1000ml/hr. Trust and organizational policy will dictate that only those trained in the use of the volumetric pump will be allowed to operate one.

Observing the patient
As with any medication it is paramount that a patient receiving an IV infusion/solution is monitored frequently. Depending on the type of medication, pulse, blood pressure, temperature and respiration should be regularly monitored throughout the infusion.

Clinical tip

Baseline observations should be made before the infusion is begun. This will allow any anomalies to be further monitored during the infusion.

Observing the cannula site
The patency of the cannula or central line must be checked prior to administration of any medications or solution. It is not a requirement to routinely withdraw blood from the device and discard it prior to flushing unless it is from a central line and is required for blood sampling. A blood sample can be obtained from a peripheral cannula at the initial siting of the cannula only – subsequent blood samples have to be taken from a different vein.

The cannula or central line should be flushed at established intervals to promote and maintain patency and to prevent the mixing of any incompatible solutions or medications.

Clinical tip

Flushing with 0.9 per cent sodium chloride to ensure patency should be performed before, between and after the administration of incompatible medications or solutions. The usual volume is between 5 and 10ml of sodium chloride.

A peripheral cannula should be removed every 72–96 hours or sooner if any infection or complications are suspected and re-sited if still required. Unused and unwanted cannulas should be removed as soon as possible to prevent the risk of an infection developing.

Observing the infusion

When nursing a patient with a central line it is important that the nurse aspirates the device to check blood return and confirm patency prior to the administration of any medication or solutions. If when aspirating the line there is an absence of blood, an attempt should be made to flush the device. If any sort of resistance is encountered then undue force should not be applied. With a peripheral cannula it may be necessary to remove the cannula completely.

Plasma and plasma substitutes

There are two common types of IV solution used in fluid replacement. The first is *colloids* such as gelofusine and haemaccel. Colloids are mainly used as plasma volume expanders in the treatment of circulatory shock (in a cardiac arrest for example). The second is *crystalloids* such as normal saline (containing the electrolytes sodium and chloride) which have a concentration of dissolved particles equal to that of the intracellular fluid. This means that the 'pressure' inside and outside the cell remains the same (isotonic). There remains a controversial debate as to the administration of crystalloids versus colloids in fluid replacement and there is evidence for both types of fluid resuscitation having a part to play in maintaining home-

ostasis. It is important to remember that as the molecules in crystalloid fluids are much smaller than those in colloids, twice the amount of fluid may be required to maintain blood pressure. In a colloid infusion, which pulls fluid into the bloodstream, the effects can last for several days.

Clinical tip

The patient's vital signs will always need to be monitored, using either method, for hypertension, dyspnoea and a bounding pulse which are all signs of hypervolaemia (fluid overload).

Colloids

Colloids have large molecules that do not readily cross capillary membranes and are retained in the blood vessels, which helps to maintain blood pressure, tissue perfusion and to stabilize circulatory haemostasis. Colloids are routinely used in situations where there is a need to maintain haemodynamic stability. Examples of colloids are albumin, plasma protein fraction, dextran and hetastarch.

Although colloids are more expensive than crystalloids, on a volume-for-volume basis they are more effective in restoring blood volume.

Crystalloids

Crystalloid solutions can freely cross the capillary wall of the cell. Sodium chloride 0.9 per cent (normal saline) provides short-term fluid replacement (30–60 minutes of blood volume replacement), because it is rapidly absorbed into the interstitial spaces as its molecules are much smaller than those of colloids. As normal saline is rapidly absorbed it is considered isotonic. As the osmotic pressure within and surrounding the cell is 0.9 per cent the fluid is compatible with replacing lost fluids within the body. Crystalloids are used successfully to replace intravascular volume and electrolytes in conditions such as diarrhoea and vomiting. To achieve full fluid replacement in blood loss the volume of normal saline to be infused must be three times the volume of blood lost. This can be detrimental in some instances where giving a large amount of fluid can put a tremendous strain on the heart. In patients with underlying cardiac problems colloids may appear to be a better choice as less fluid is needed to achieve a similar outcome.

Another common crystalloid is glucose 5 per cent in water. Due to the fact that glucose metabolizes quickly it acts like a hypotonic solution and leaves water behind. This is especially important as it can cause renal impairment and cardiac problems due to fluid overload. It is important not to infuse large quantities of glucose 5 per cent as this may lead to hyperglycaemia (too much sugar in the blood). Lastly, Ringer's solution is considered to be isotonic as it contains all the compounds found in the extracellular space: sodium, potassium, calcium and chloride.

Using any colloid or crystalloid infusion has a benefit to the patient, albeit a short to medium amount of support time. However, if neither crystalloids nor colloids are effective in treating imbalances, especially during blood loss, then the patient may require a blood transfusion. Colloid and crystalloid therapy certainly has its place in supporting homeostasis for the patient while cross-matching the patient's blood.

Once cross-matching has occurred, if blood is to be transfused then this is achieved via a blood administration set with an integral mesh filter. Standard blood administration sets already contain in-line filters that will remove unwanted particles from the transfused blood.

Nursing observations

Nurses overseeing an infusion of plasma must remain vigilant for any potential complications that may arise from infusing large volumes of fluid. Patients receiving replacement fluids can develop fluid-induced hypothermia (the patient gets very cold due to the amount of fluid being administered, which can reduce the core temperature to below 37 degrees), hypocalcaemia (decreased calcium), hyperkalaemia (increased potassium), clotting problems and experience disturbances with their acid/base balance. As with any introduction of a fluid the patient should be observed within the first few minutes to ensure that no allergic reaction is evident.

> **Clinical tip**
>
> If a reaction should occur the nurse should stop the fluids immediately and seek medical assistance.

Patients should receive regular observation of their blood pressure, temperature, pulse, respiration and general mental state. The timing of the nursing observations may depend on the patient's age and medical condition.

As there are so many important aspects to consider during the administration of fluids, nurses should have a thorough working knowledge of the relevant principles and applications surrounding fluid therapy and be able to exercise their professional judgement at all times.

Nutritional support

Nutritional support should be considered for any patient who is unable to eat their usual dietary requirements. Medical conditions that may affect nutritional intake include diarrhoea and sickness, ulcerative colitis, pancreatitis, bowel surgery (including time to rest the bowel) and peritonitis. Patients suffering these conditions may not be meeting the body's calorific requirements to produce enough energy for everyday activities.

There are a variety of ways to meet nutritional requirements such as protein supplements, vitamin and mineral supplements, modification of diet, gastroscopy (percutaneous endoscopically placed gastrostomy (PEG)) and enteral tube feeding (nasogastric/nasoduodenal/nasojejunal).

Nasogastric tubes

Intubation using a nasogastric (NG) tube involves inserting a plastic tube through the nose, past the throat and into the stomach. The stomach then acts as a reservoir to hold and release the food at a steady rate. A positive benefit from this type of tube placement is that the stomach still produces the acidic environment which destroys potential bacteria within the food. Feeding via NG tubes is usually on a short-term basis, generally more than five days but less than four weeks.

Contraindications

Intubation of this kind is contraindicated in patients with base of skull fractures, any type of facial fractures (especially to the nose) and any form of obstructed airway. NG tubes are also contraindicated in bariatric procedures (e.g. gastric bypass/bands). The risk of aspiration is high but can be minimized by feeding patients sat up at an angle of 30–45 degrees, and keeping them sat up for at least 30 minutes after the feed is complete.

Nasojejunal tubes

Like the NG tube a nasojejunal tube is passed via the nose. The difference is that the tube is advanced beyond the oesophagogastric and pyloric sphincters into the jejunum (small intestine between the duodenum and the ileum). This has the benefit of reducing the risk of aspiration. However, because the tube has bypassed the acidic environment of the stomach, which is now not acting as an acidic reservoir, the feed itself needs to be sterile and delivered at a slower rate, giving the small intestine time to assimilate the food. This type of feeding is especially beneficial to unconscious patients who need to be nursed flat.

Percutaneous endoscopic gastrostomy

This type of tube passes directly through the abdominal wall into the stomach or the jejunum and is ideally suited for patients who require long-term feeding – for example, stroke patients who have difficulty swallowing. Percutaneous endoscopic gastrostomy (PEG) feeding carries a risk of aspiration, so the patient should remain at an angle of 30–45 degrees during feeding.

Enteral feed (within the GI tract)

This type of feed is completely influenced by the patient's nutritional requirements and GI function. The content of this type of feed is in itself nutritionally complete. The feed contains fluid, electrolytes, vitamins, trace elements, energy and protein and is mostly in liquid form. Enteral feeds are usually made up with the advice of a dietician who has assessed the patient's nutritional status and calorific intake.

Parenteral feed (not via the GI tract)

Parenteral nutrition is delivered via a central venous catheter with the result that the greatest risk to the patient is infection. Therefore catheter insertion is by aseptic technique, and it is important that administration sets are changed every 24 hours. To administer the accurate delivery of a parenteral feed a volumetric infusion pump is used. Any patient likely to be 'nil by mouth' for longer than five days should be considered for a parenteral feed if enteral nutrition is not able to be established.

Case studies

① Simon is a 50-year-old who has been knocked off a powerful motorbike by a lorry at 50mph. He has sustained an open fracture to his left femur (thigh bone) and a number of lacerations to his hands and face. On arrival at A&E his blood pressure is 90/45mmHg, pulse 125bpm and respirations 25rpm. In progress, via a peripheral cannula, is an IV infusion of gelofusine (a colloid). Simon appears pale, clammy, confused and disorientated and is seen to be visibly shaking. Your mentor asks you to explain to her why he is being given gelofusine as opposed to 0.9 per cent normal saline (crystalloid). She also asks you to comment on his vital signs and visual cues.

- Why is a colloid being administered rather than a crystalloid in this instance?
- What do Simon's vital signs and symptoms tell you about his overall medical condition?

② An 85-year-old severely dehydrated patient has an IV infusion of 0.9 per cent normal saline running via a peripheral cannula sited in the back of her wrist. She rings her bell and complains that her hand is swollen and uncomfortable. On inspection you notice that the back of her hand appears quite pale and the IV flow rate is very slow. Her hand appears to show tightness around the cannula site and is also very cold to the touch.

- What do you think might have happened in this instance?
- What should you do about it?

Key learning points

Introduction

➤ One of the most important aspects of a nurse's job is the administration of prescribed medication. This may take the form of IV medication/solutions.

Anatomy and physiology

➤ The walls of all blood vessels, arteries and veins are composed of three layers of tissue called tunica.

Veins used in intravenous therapy

➤ There are commonly used veins for peripheral and central venous therapy.

Fluid compartments

➤ About 25 litres of water is selectively stored within cells (intracellular).
➤ Extracellular fluid (fluid that surrounds the cells) makes about 18 litres.
➤ In infancy there is a greater storage percentage of body water in the interstitial spaces than in adults.

Fluid types

➤ These include isotonic, hypotonic and hypertonic solutions.

Fluid balance

➤ A person's daily intake and output of fluid is approximately 2600ml.
➤ Fluid loss is divided into two groups: sensible and insensible.

Electrolytes

➤ There are seven main electrolytes which are a major component of body fluids.

→

←

Fluid and electrolyte imbalances

➢ These include dehydration, increase in temperature, loss of whole blood, loss of plasma and bleeding disorders.

Intravenous infusion

➢ Commonly called a 'drip' because the method of delivery employs a drip chamber which prevents air entering the body.
➢ This is the fastest way to deliver fluid and blood transfusions. It is also used to correct electrolyte imbalances, alleviate dehydration and administer medications.

Risks

➢ Any breach or break in the skin's integrity carries an element of risk of infection.
➢ If bacteria get into the bloodstream the infection is likely to be septicaemia which can have life-threatening consequences.

Preparation and procedure

➢ IV medication should ideally be checked with two registrants or in exceptional circumstances the registrant and another competent person prior to its administration.
➢ Prior to administration a nurse's responsibility should be to appropriately label any containers, vials and syringes; identify the correct patient; ensure all checks for allergies, content, dose, rate and route have been made and that any expiry date is thoroughly adhered to.

Infusion systems

➢ Gravity flow infusion devices are often used when there is no precedent to deliver a precise regimen of a fluid/drug in an exact amount of time.
➢ Volumetric pumps work via a linear peristaltic pumping mechanism.

Observing the patient

➢ Depending on the type of medication being infused, regular pulse, blood pressure, temperature and respiration rates should be measured throughout the infusion.

Observing the infusion

➢ The patency of either the cannula or central line must be checked prior to administration of any medications or solution.

Plasma and plasma substitutes

➢ Colloids are mainly used as plasma volume expanders in the treatment of circulatory shock (in a cardiac arrest for example).
➢ Crystalloids such as normal saline have a concentration of dissolved particles equal to that of the intracellular fluid.

Nursing observations

➤ Nurses overseeing an infusion of fluids must remain vigilant for any potential complications that may arise.
➤ The patient should be observed within the first few minutes to ensure no allergic reaction is evident.

Nutritional support

➤ Intubation using an NG means inserting a plastic tube through the nose, past the throat and into the stomach.
➤ A nasojejunal tube is passed via the nose in the same way. The difference is that the tube is advanced beyond the oesophagogastric and pyloric sphincters into the jejunum.
➤ In PEG a tube passes directly through the abdominal wall into the stomach or the jejunum.
➤ Parenteral nutrition describes IV administration of nutritional support.

Calculations

1 How many ml are in 0.455L?
2 The total volume to be given is 1200ml. The time over which this is to be given is four hours. How many ml per hour would you give?
3 The total volume to be given is 120ml. The time over which this is to be given is two hours. How many ml per hour would you give?
4 The total volume to be given is 90ml. The time over which this is to be given is 45 minutes. The drop factor is 20. How many drops per minute will be delivered?
5 The total volume to be given is 960ml. The time over which this is to be given is 24 hours. The drop factor is 15. How many drops per minute will be delivered?
6 The total volume to be given is 1200ml. The time over which this is to be given is eight hours. The drop factor is 60. How many drops per minute will be delivered?
7 1.5L of normal saline is required to be given over four hours. Using a giving set which delivers 10 drops/ml how many drops per minute will need to be given?
8 The volume remaining is 600ml. The drop factor on the set is 20. The drops per minute (calculated when set up) is 40. How many minutes will this take to deliver?
9 1L of IV fluids is charted over 11 hours. The drop factor is 10. The IV has been running for 9 hours and 45 minutes. 100ml remain. How many drops per minute are needed so that the IV finishes in the required time?
10 The volume remaining is 420ml. The drop factor on the set is 20. The drops per minute (calculated when set up) is 84. How many minutes will this take?

For further assistance with calculations, please see Meriel Hutton's book *Essential Calculation Skills for Nurses, Midwives and Healthcare Practitioners* (Open University Press 2009).

Multiple choice questions

1 The most commonly used veins for peripheral venous therapy are

a) External jugular vein
b) Metacarpal vein
c) Left subclavian vein
d) Superior vena cava

2 On average how much water does the average adult body contain?

a) 30–39L
b) 40–45L
c) 50–55L
d) 60+L

3 An isotonic solution is

a) 10% dextrose
b) 0.45% saline
c) Dextrose 2.5% in water
d) Normal saline 0.9%

4 Colloids are

a) Balanced salt solutions that can freely cross the capillary wall of the cell
b) Short-term fluid replacements
c) Large molecules that do not readily cross capillary membranes
d) Used to replace intravascular volume and electrolytes

5 Nasojejunal intubation means that the tube is sitting in

a) The duodenum
b) The stomach
c) The gall bladder
d) Part of the small intestine

6 Patients receiving replacement fluid therapy can develop

a) Hypothermia
b) Hypocalcaemia
c) Hyperkalaemia
d) All of the above

7 A peripheral cannula should be relocated

a) Every 2–3 days
b) Every 7 days
c) Every 4 days
d) Every 24 hours

8 Insensible fluid losses occur through

a) Urination
b) Vomit
c) Sweating
d) Wound exudates

9 Your patient develops warmth, swelling, pain, increased temperature and redness around the peripheral IV cannula site. What is likely to be causing it?

a) Infiltration
b) Occlusion
c) Phlebitis
d) Extravasation

10 What is the maximum amount of time that TPN solutions are permitted to infuse before the bag must be replaced?

a) 24 hours
b) 48 hours
c) 12 hours
d) 16 hours

Recommended further reading

Barber, P. and Robertson, D. (2012) *Essentials of Pharmacology for Nurses*, 2nd edn. Maidenhead: Open University Press.

Beckwith, S. and Franklin, P. (2007) *Oxford Handbook of Nurse Prescribing*. Oxford: Oxford University Press.

Brenner, G.M. and Stevens, C.W. (2009) *Pharmacology*, 3rd edn. Philadelphia, PA: Saunders Elsevier.

Clayton, B.D. (2009) *Basic Pharmacology for Nurses*, 15th edn. St Louis, MO: Mosby Elsevier.

Coben, D. and Atere-Roberts, E. (2005) *Calculations for Nursing and Healthcare*, 2nd edn. Basingstoke: Palgrave Macmillan.

Downie, G., Mackenzie, J. and Williams, A. (2007) *Pharmacology and Medicines Management for Nurses*, 4th edn. Edinburgh: Churchill Livingstone.

Gatford, J.D. and Phillips, N. (2006) *Nursing Calculations*, 7th edn. Edinburgh: Churchill Livingstone Elsevier.

Greenstein, B. (2009) *Clinical Pharmacology for Nurses*, 18th edn. Edinburgh: Churchill Livingstone.

Hutton, M. (2009) *Essential Calculation Skills for nurses, Midwives and Healthcare Practitioners.* Maidenhead: Open University Press.

Karch, A.M. (2008) *Focus on Nursing Pharmacology*, 4th edn. Philadelphia, PA: Lippincott Williams & Wilkins.

Lapham, R. and Agar, H. (2009) *Drug Calculations for Nurses: A Step-by-step Approach*, 3rd edn. London: Arnold.

National Safety Patient Agency (2010) *Patient Safety: Observatory Safety in Doses; Medication Safety Incidents in the NHS (2007 and 2009)*, www.npsa.nhs.uk.

NICE (National Institute for Health and Clinical Excellence) (2010) Nutrition support for adults oral nutrition support, enteral tube feeding and parenteral nutrition, www.nice.org.uk/nicemedia/live/10978/29981/29981.pdf.

NMC (Nursing and Midwifery Council) (2007) *Standard for Medicine Management*, www.nmc-uk.org/Publications/Standards.

Royal College of Nursing (2010) *Standards for Administration of IV Therapy*, www.rcn.org.uk.

Simonson, T., Aarbakke, J., Kay, I., Coleman, I., Sinnott, P. and Lyssa, R. (2006) *Illustrated Pharmacology for Nurses*. London: Hodder Arnold.

Starkings, S. and Krause, L. (2010) *Passing Calculation Tests for Nursing Students*. Exeter: Learning Matters.

United Kingdom Medicines Information (2010) *United Kingdom Injectable Medicines Guide*, http://ukmi.nhs.uk.

Medicines used on the skin

8

Chapter contents

Learning objectives

After studying this chapter you should be able to:

- Briefly outline the structure and function of the body surface.
- Understand the concept of true topical, topical systemic and topical invasive medicines in relation to the routes of medicines used for skin disorders.
- Demonstrate, by giving examples, an understanding of what is meant by a 'vehicle' in relation to the delivery of drugs to the body surface.
- Define what is meant by the term 'true topical medicine'.
- Outline medicines and preparations used in keeping the body surface healthy.
- Explain the treatment options for dealing with dry and itchy skin.
- List common infestations of the hair and skin.
- Describe some of the treatments for dealing with common infestations.
- List some of the medicines used in treating warts.
- Demonstrate an understanding of the terms 'eczema', 'psoriasis' and 'acne vulgaris'.
- Discuss the various treatment options for dealing with the disorders eczema, psoriasis and acne.
- Use basic maths in order to calculate simple drug dosages.

Introduction

The original title for this chapter was 'Topical medicines'. A process of reflection made it apparent that, on the whole, the use of the term 'topical' in medical literature has not kept pace with advances in our understanding of the surface of the body as a means of drug application, nor the more sophisticated preparations available. The true meaning of the term 'topical' has become blurred over time, and no two books seem to address the subject in the same way. Some include a chapter on 'topical' medicines; others refer to the 'topical route'. Still others talk about 'topical' as a *form* of medicine, for example, a 'topical powder' or a 'topical steroid'. The term 'topical' is frequently used when 'transdermal', 'percutaneous' (through the skin) or 'transmucosal' would be more accurate.

This chapter aims to take a fresh approach to the consideration of the term 'topical'. For comprehensive coverage, the term has been subdivided into three categories: *true topical, topical systemic* and *topical invasive*. Each category depends on the location of application and whether the effect is *local* or *systemic*. The bulk of the chapter focuses on 'true

topical' medicines, considering those preparations applied to the body surface either to keep it healthy or to treat a variety of conditions.

The term 'topical medicine' is one to which it is difficult to give a precise and accurate meaning. The pharmacological use of the term 'topical' is often used interchangeably with the word 'local'. Generally this refers to the route of administration of a drug that is applied directly to the part of the body being treated. Historically, it meant 'accessible areas of the body surface', mainly the skin (cutaneous application). In its initial and truest sense, this may be thought of as 'true topical' in that the preparations work *exactly* where they are put; they do not cross through the skin surface, exerting only a local effect. The skin was considered to be such an effective barrier that drugs would not be absorbed through it.

Other accessible areas of the body's surface include the hair, nails and mucous membranes. These were, and still are, used to treat a variety of conditions, infections and infestations 'topically'. Preparations have even been used on the body surface for embalming after death.

Preparations may also be applied 'topically' to keep the area healthy, and to prevent disease. This notion of prevention may well be underestimated in pharmacology. In its simplest form, examples include the application of cosmetics and moisturising agents to the skin, a salve to a burn, or witch hazel to a bruise. Although not thought of as 'medicines', many proprietary insect repellents work in such a way, preventing the insect from landing on the skin. If an insect does not land, it cannot bite, and irritation and infection cannot occur. The key phrase here is 'affecting only the area to which it is applied' – an insect will happily bite an area *adjacent* to that where repellent has been applied.

These are examples of what can be considered true topical medicines because they work where they are put, they do not have to cross any barriers or membranes. Smaller doses can be used than if the drug was given via the oral or enteral route (via the digestive tract), making these medicines correspondingly safer. A major advantage of the parenteral (non-digestive) administration of drugs is that they bypass the liver, avoiding the 'first pass effect' (see Barber and Robertson 2012: Chapter 1).

An important clinical point is that, in certain circumstances, some potent drugs considered as 'true topical' can, to a certain extent, be absorbed into the bloodstream. They can also be stored in the skin and hair, which act as a reservoir, causing potentially toxic side-effects. As will be seen later, one example is topical steroids and another is the drug pilocarpine. Applied as drops to the eye, Pilocarpine constricts the pupil and aids drainage. Shortly after application, however, the drug may pass through nearby structures and enter the general circulation, possibly resulting in unwanted effects such as dizziness, incoherence and headache. Although unpleasant, these may be very short-lived, and the beneficial effects last much longer. Nevertheless, this raises further practical considerations in our understanding of what we consider to *be* topical drugs, an increasing number of which (such as antimicrobials and steroids) can now be sold over the counter. This places greater emphasis on the need for both consumers and carers to understand their appropriate use and application.

Many preparations applied to the skin or mucous membranes are *not* true topical. They are designed to behave very differently, as they do not treat directly the part to which they have been applied. In the last 40 years advances in biology and pharmacology have made it possible for drugs to be developed which are able to cross through the natural barrier of the skin or mucous membrane surface, finding their way via a local capillary into the general circulation and exerting their effects in other parts of the body.

These medicines retain some of the characteristics considered under the 'topical' umbrella. They are applied locally to accessible areas of the body surface but, because they exert their effect systemically, might be thought of as 'topical systemic'. When drugs are formulated to cross through the skin they are called *transdermal*; when crossing through a mucous membrane, the term used is *transmucosal*. Both may be considered as topical systemic routes – topical in that they are applied locally, systemic because the drugs are absorbed for subsequent systemic action. Examples include skin patches for hormone replacement therapy (HRT) and tablets of glyceryl trinitrate (GTN) placed under the tongue for angina.

In some circumstances, the same route can be used for both true topical and 'topical systemic' purposes. One such example is inhalation. Drugs inhaled to treat asthma work locally on the airways (true topical) but the target tissue for inhaled volatile anaesthetics is the brain, an example of the topical systemic route.

It is also now possible to make use of invasive techniques. Certain drugs are injected directly to previously inaccessible areas, enabling them to exert a local action. Because they exert their action where they are put, such treatments are topical in the true sense of the word. The use of invasive technique, however, means such treatments may be more accurately described as 'topical invasive'. Corticosteroids, for example, can be delivered directly into a joint to treat arthritis, and antibiotics can be injected into the pleural space to treat a local infection. Such invasive methods can still accurately be described as topical because the drug has been applied to the area being treated. In the original meaning of the term, however, that area is not readily accessible. The most important principle of local application and action nevertheless still applies. This method retains the benefits of a local action and is an area of pharmacology which has developed rapidly in recent years.

In order to understand how the preparations presented exert their effect, an understanding of the relevant structure and function of the body surface is required.

Structure and function of the body surface

The surface of the body is made up of skin, skin derivatives or appendages (hair and nails) and is continuous with the membranes covering the eye and ear and lining the mouth, rectum, vagina and respiratory structures. Together with the sweat and oil glands, these make up the *integumentory system* which keeps us intact and plays a major role in homeostasis. The tissue making up the skin and mucous membranes is called *epithelium*, itself made up of several different types of epithelial cells, arranged in single or multiple layers. Epithelial cells differ according to the structures they cover and the job they have to do. Some are very complex.

> **Clinical tip**
>
> Alterations in the normal development and functioning of the structures involved can affect, to a greater or lesser extent, the overall well-being of an individual. Skin problems are common in all age groups and can be helped by a range of true topical preparations, many of which address the altered physiology causing the problem.

The skin

Often taken for granted, the skin is a large, complex and multifunctional organ that forms approx-

imately 16 per cent of our body weight. It provides the boundary that separates us from our outside environment and enables us to function within it. This two-way anatomical barrier prevents water and harmful substances entering the body, while excreting excess water and many waste products (including some drugs) in sweat.

Skin protects the underlying tissues and organs from external factors such as heat and chemicals. It contains secretions that can kill harmful microorganisms while its pigmentation provides a defence against potentially damaging ultraviolet (UV) light. Acting as a reservoir for blood, it synthesizes vitamin D (essential for calcium absorption from the gut and its mobilization from the bones) from sunlight, and provides a means of social and sexual communication.

> **Clinical tip**
>
> If we consider everything that the skin has to do on a daily basis, it is not difficult to appreciate the wide variety of problems that can occur when normal processes go wrong.

Skin compartments

When describing the skin three distinct parts are generally considered:

- The epidermis
- The dermis
- The underlying connective tissues, often referred to as the subcutis or hypodermis

It must be remembered, however, that this distinction is for study purposes only, they function as a whole. Their relationship is illustrated in Figure 8.1.

The epidermis

The outer, thinner compartment of the skin is called the *epidermis*. It is made from four layers (strata) of squamous (scaly) epithelium and

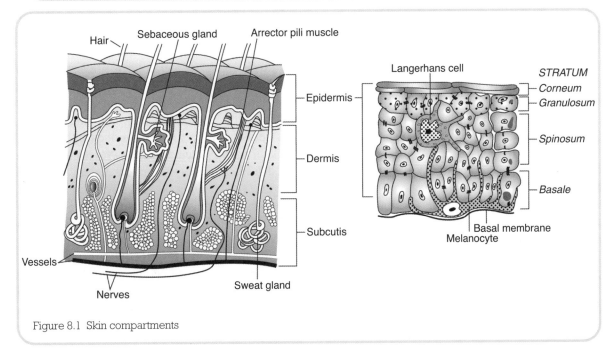

Figure 8.1 Skin compartments

contains a number of different functioning cells. These are formed in the deeper (basal) layer, moving gradually to the top layer, losing their nucleus and becoming progressively impregnated with a hard, protective protein called keratin as they go, before being shed from the body. The epidermis has no blood supply of its own, relying on nutrients passing up from arterial vessels in the dermis and waste materials, apart from sweat, moving down to be collected by venous and lymphatic vessels. It contains a variety of enzyme systems capable of a number of functions, including drug biotransformation. The normal process of maturation and shredding is called *orthokeratosis*. No one is sure how long this process takes; a month, 50 or 70 days have all been suggested. If, however, it goes wrong at any stage it can create a number of skin problems (e.g. in the skin disorder psoriasis, orthokeratosis is reduced to 8–10 days). Depending on the nature of the disordered physiology, these problems will require true topical medication.

The dermis

Also called the *stratum basale, basement membrane* or *Malpighian layer* this is the deepest layer of the epidermis. It is composed of a single layer of columnar-shaped cells forming an irregular ridged surface (the ridges are called *rete ridges*) which forms the border between the epidermis and dermis, anchoring them together during foetal development. The patterns of the ridges are formed in the dermis and are different in every individual, creating our distinct fingerprint.

The basal layer mostly contains the skin's stem cells, *keratinocytes*. Undergoing cell division only in this layer (usually during sleep) these enable the epidermis to continually reproduce itself. As each cell divides, one daughter cell remains in the basal layer, the other moving upwards through the other layers of the epidermis. As the keratinocyte moves up, it begins to lose its chemistry and gradually dies.

Cells which produce the dark pigment melanin (melanocytes) are also found in the basal layer, the exception being the skin on the palms and soles. Melanin absorbs energy from UV radiation. Acting as a scavenging system, its production is stimulated by sunlight. Melanocytes are therefore more abundant in areas of skin exposed to the sun. Specialized *Merkel cells*, sensitive to touch, are also found here. This layer changes significantly with ageing.

The subcutis

This layer is also referred to as the *stratum spinosum* and is 8 to 10 cells thick. Most of the living epidermal keratinocytes which have moved up from the basal layer are found here. Keratinocytes become joined to each other by protrusions that look like intercellular bridges or 'prickles' before undergoing a series of changes which destroy the cell nucleus. The cells become flattened as they move towards the surface. The keratinocytes take in protective melanin by phagocytosis (digestion). Langerhans cells are also found here. These play an important part in digesting bacteria and other foreign materials, providing, together with various chemicals, mast and other white cells (including T cell), immune support.

The granular layer

Also known as the *stratum granulosum*, the cells in this layer begin to make keratin. The nucleus in each cell also disintegrates here, thus they can no longer divide. The cell structure is replaced with a tough layer of keratin. A fifth layer of clear, flat, dead cells can be found between the stratum corneum and the granular layer, but only on the palms of the hands and soles of the feet because these areas need to be thicker and tougher. This layer is not needed elsewhere.

The stratum corneum

Some books refer to this as the *cornified layer*. Knowledge of its structure and function is very important for the practical use and application of true topical and topical systemic drugs as it is to this layer that they are applied. The stratum corneum is the 'gate-keeping' and 'rate-limiting' water resistant barrier through which drugs must penetrate if they are to exert both a local and systemic action. Consisting of tough (though still flexible) flattened, dead cells and completely filled with keratin, it is the end result of the keratinization process which began in the deeper layers. The keratinocytes contain a substance that helps them to retain water – a natural, built-in moisturising factor which aids the pliability and elasticity of skin. The stratum corneum can be thought of as a brick wall with strong, intact layers of bricks made of keratin held together by a 'mortar' of fatty glue-like substance made of ceramides, cholesterol and free fatty acids (lipids) (see Figure 8.2). These intercellular lipids bind the keratinocytes together and stop them from drying out (desiccating). This helps the cells to swell, reducing the risk of cracks forming between them. Protein structures called *desmosomes* act like rivets, holding the cells together. *Urea* is an important physiological factor in helping to regulate the water-binding capacity in the skin, and it has been demonstrated that a urea deficit is present in some skin diseases.

A feedback mechanism in the outer skin controls normal shedding, allowing the right amount of skin to be shed at the right time. The stratum corneum *chymotrypic enzyme* helps to break down keratinocytes, while an inhibitor slows down the process.

The protein *filaggrin* is also present, having an essential role in the skin barrier function. As a further chemical protection against harmful microorganisms the skin has an 'acid mantle' with a pH of 5.5.

Cell adhesion and the molecules facilitating it are of great importance for healthy skin. A range of dermatological disorders have been identified as being caused when this process breaks down. Breaking this barrier exposes the underlying tissues and organs to mechanical damage, dehydration, microbial invasion and temperature variation.

Mucous membranes

Moist *mucous membranes* (also called *mucosa*) line many structures and cavities that open to the exterior (mouth, nose, lungs, eyes, anus, ears and vagina). Although made of epithelium, they contain no keratin and provide an excellent site for the absorption of drugs.

Glands

Sebaceous glands secrete an oily substance, *sebum*, supplying water resistance and lubrication to

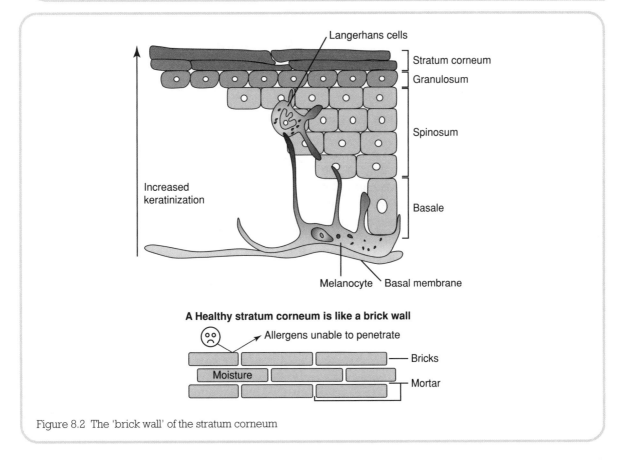

Figure 8.2 The 'brick wall' of the stratum corneum

the skin and hair. Although part of the epidermis they penetrate down into the dermis where there is a rich supply of capillary vessels, providing oxygen and nutrients.

Sweat or *sudiferous* glands are of two main types: *eccrine* and *apocrine*. Found practically everywhere on the body surface (apart from lips and genitals), eccrine glands are most numerous on the palms of the hands and soles of the feet. Beginning in the dermis, they extend to the epidermis as a long coiled duct opening on the surface of an epidermal pore. This duct is surrounded by a ring of keratin, and is easily blocked by inflammation or even hydration. Apocrine sweat glands are found mainly in the skin of the axilla, nipples, outer ear, eyelids and the perianal and genital areas. Found in the ear, *ceruminous* glands secrete a waxy substance which, mixing with sebum, forms cerumen or ear wax. This traps foreign particles in the ear canal, preventing them from entering the ear.

Hair

Hair (also known as *pili*) is composed of welded dead keratinized cells. A hair consists of a shaft above the surface, a root penetrating the dermis and subcutaneous layer and a hair follicle surrounding the root. Hair on the head protects against the sun's rays.

Nails

Protecting our fingertips and toes and made of hard keratinous cells packed tightly together, nails have three main parts to their structure. The visible part is the main body growing over the end of the finger or toe. The nail *root* and the nail *matrix* are hidden, and are concerned with transforming superficial cells into nail cells.

The dermis

Thicker than the epidermis, the dermis (or true skin) protects the underlying muscles, bones and organs. Its thickness varies greatly, being thinnest in the eyelids and thickest on the palms of the hands and soles of the feet. It has two parts: the outer papillary dermis (the unique convoluted pattern forming a fingerprint), and a looser, coarse-fibred reticular layer containing bundles of collagen and elastin fibres which anchor the skin to the fat-rich subcutaneous tissue (hypodermis). Blood vessels, lymph vessels, white blood cells, tactile and other nerves, smooth muscles and a variety of special glands are also found here.

The hypodermis or subcutis
Underlying the deepest layer of the dermis, loose connective areolar tissue and varying amounts of fat are found here.

Factors affecting the skin barrier

Having immature skin barriers, the very young (those under 6 months of age) and pre-term babies are particularly at risk of having very dry skin, especially where there is a family history of skin problems. Later in life, skin changes often result in dry skin and loss of skin integrity. The epidermis thins and the keratinocytes do not adhere to each other as well. This reduces their water retention ability, weakening their barrier function. In addition, fewer Langerhans cells are produced, weakening the ability of the skin to protect itself against invading micro-organisms and allergens. Ageing skin has a thinner dermis, is prone to damage and has a slower healing time than younger skin. There is also a reduction in hair follicles which can impede drug delivery. All these factors have implications for the use of true topical preparations which will be seen later in the chapter.

Clinical tip

When incontinence exposes the skin to urine and faeces it can cause it to soften and over-hydrate, making the barrier function less robust. Excessive damp and warmth in body creases can encourage fungal and bacterial invasion and a breakdown of the skin barrier.

Drug absorption and the body surface

Molecules can penetrate the skin by three routes: through the stratum corneum, the sweat ducts or the sebaceous follicles. The degree to which a drug intended for both true topical and topical systemic use will work depends on the inherent potency of the drug and its ability to penetrate the layers of the epidermis (lipid solubility). Once a drug has crossed the epidermis it can pass easily through the dermis, and drugs formulated for systemic (percutaneous) absorption pass into the capillaries. Percutaneous absorption necessitates passage through the epidermis, the papillary dermis and then into the bloodstream.

The biological 'brick wall' of the stratum corneum must be overcome if drugs are to cross through it. Lipid-soluble substances can pass through the 'mortar' more easily than water-soluble ones. Pharmaceutical companies carefully formulate preparations so that they can reach and work only where they are needed. The *active ingredients* are designed to be able to variously:

- remain on the skin surface (e.g. cleansing agents, sunscreens, insect repellents, antimicrobials and cosmetics);
- be absorbed to different layers of the skin along a concentration gradient (e.g. in the treatment of skin disorders);
- diffuse across the epidermis (transdermal) or mucosa (transmucosal) and freely permeate underlying structures into the systemic circulation.

In contrast to the absorption of oral drugs which are almost completely absorbed within a few hours, drugs applied to the skin have a poor and slow rate of absorption. They can, however, be used in much smaller concentrations than those given orally, and avoid the first pass effect in the liver.

> **Clinical tip**
>
> The ability of a drug to cross the stratum corneum depends not only on its lipid solubility but also on the *integrity* of the skin surface. Damaged, abraded or eczematized skin provides less of a barrier. It is important to be aware of this when applying medicines to the skin.

Other factors influencing the rate of absorption include the thickness of the stratum corneum (which varies in different parts of the body), the concentration of the medication, the frequency of application and patient concordance. The most penetrable areas are the mucous membranes. Absorption through these can be very rapid because they have no outer keratinized layer and the nearby dermis has an excellent blood supply, freely open for drugs to pass through.

The most penetrable areas of the skin in descending order are:

- the scrotum
- the eyelids
- the face
- the chest and back
- the upper arms and legs
- the dorsa of the hands and feet
- the palms and plantar skin
- the nails

Solvents, surfactants and alcohols in preparations applied to the skin can damage the keratinocytes, increasing penetration and therefore absorption. Hair enhances penetration and therefore the scalp and beard pose less of a barrier. It is

important to remember that the skin may also act as a reservoir for drugs.

> **Clinical tip**
>
> The stratum corneum in older people is thinner and also poorly hydrated. There is also a reduction in hair follicles which impedes drug delivery. The skin of neonates absorbs local medicines more efficiently. This is important to remember when applying a true topical preparation.

Occlusion

The absorption of some drugs can be enhanced (10 to 100 times) through *occlusion*, the use of closed airtight dressings or greasy ointment bases which increase hydration and the temperature of the stratum corneum. Occlusion can lead to more rapid onset of drugs and increased efficacy (e.g. in local anaesthetics). It may also lead to a more rapid appearance of adverse effects such as thinning of the skin due to steroid therapy. Occlusion may promote infections such as *folliculitis* or *miliaria*, and is contraindicated for use with non-steroidal anti-inflammatory drugs (NSAIDs) or rubefacients.

Occlusion techniques include:

- application under an airtight dressing;
- use of cotton gloves or socks.

Vehicles used to deliver drugs to the surface of the body

Any medication applied to the body surface, whether for local or for systemic purposes, must be incorporated into an appropriate *vehicle* or *base*. This enables it, once applied, to remain in place long enough for it to penetrate at least the superficial cells of the stratum corneum. Here it subsequently releases the active ingredient into the pharmacologically relevant compartment of the skin.

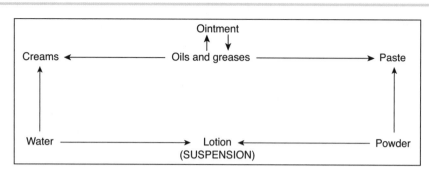

Figure 8.3 Composition of vehicles

Composition of vehicles

Skin preparations make use of many different vehicle types: liquids, greases and powders mixed in various combinations to produce creams, ointments, lotions, gels and pastes (see Figure 8.3).

As well as providing a base to incorporate an active drug, vehicles are often used without any active substance, allowing a moisture-retaining and softening effect on dry skin. Emollients and moisturizers are particularly important in keeping the skin healthy, and are considered in detail later in the chapter.

Clinical tip

The preparation chosen will depend on the consistency required and its proposed purpose. Choosing the most appropriate vehicle is as important as the choice of drug it contains.

The choice of vehicle and drug will be influenced by:

- the severity of the problem requiring treatment;
- the sites involved;
- the personal profile and preferences of the patient.

Five main vehicle bases have been classified.

- **Hydrocarbon bases**, including hard and soft paraffin (paraffin is made from distilling wood, coal or petroleum).

- **Fats and fixed oil bases** such as olive, arachis or coconut oils.
- **Emulsifying bases.** Because these emulsify with water, they are used as soap substitutes (e.g. lanolin – hydrous wool fat). Such bases are useful for keeping active ingredients in contact with the skin for as long as possible.
- **Water-soluble bases.** These are easily washed off and are used as lubricants, to dress burns and to help drugs cross through the epidermis more readily.
- **Absorption bases** such as lanolin and beeswax.

Clinical tip

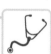

Substances called *excipients* (generally pharmacologically inert substances) may be added to a vehicle as a carrier or stabilizer for the active drug and to bulk up formulations that contain very potent active ingredients allowing for convenient and accurate dosage. The excipients contained in each topical preparation are given in the British National Formulary (BNF).

Creams and ointments

Considered as separate vehicles, creams or ointments may be used on their own, as emollients or as vehicles for active ingredients such as steroids and antimicrobials.

Clinical tip

The distinction between an ointment and a cream is not always obvious, so be careful when reading the prescription. Some preparations, neither creams nor ointments, are now available which ideally have the advantages of both.

Creams

Creams (emulsions where preparations of fine droplets of one liquid are dispersed in another) are perhaps the most commonly used and pre-scribed vehicles. Semi-solid in nature, they are intended for application to the skin or mucous membranes.

Liquids which make up creams are either aque-ous (oil or grease dispersed in water), or oily (wa-ter dispersed in oil). These are based on petroleum or lanolin, zinc cream being an example. Oil-in-water emulsions are commonly used for topical steroid products. Creams can be prepared by vary-ing the proportion of water and grease. Standard aqueous cream is composed of 70 per cent wa-ter and 30 per cent grease. Generally speaking, the higher the proportion of grease in the cream base, the more 'oily' or 'thick' the cream will be. Creams are easy to apply, easily absorbed, cross through the stratum corneum well and vanish rel-atively quickly. Since they contain water, preserva-tives must be added, and such additions may result in some patients finding creams irritating when ap-plied to damaged skin. Application may also lead to allergic contact dermatitis. Conversely, as a re-sult of water in the cream evaporating from the applied area, creams can be soothing and cooling. Creams do not rub off onto clothing, and are more acceptable to people than ointments, especially for use on the hands and feet.

There is considerable variation in ingredients, composition, pH and tolerance among generic brands, and the storage of cream preparations needs care. Instructions given for use often neglect to advise on this. Too warm and humid an environ-ment may encourage the growth of bacteria and fungi. If too dry, the cream may desicate.

Ointments

Thicker than creams, with varied bases, ointments are greasy, semi-solid preparations which may or may not be medicated. They can have water-soluble, emulsifying and non-emulsifying bases. Those which are water soluble do not stain. Emul-sifying bases aid spreading, and non-emulsifying bases (e.g. paraffin) make up the very greasy oint-ments good for a number of chronic skin diseases.

Choice of ointment base is affected by:

- Penetrability
- Stability
- Solvent property
- Irritant effects
- Ease of application and removal

Ointments can be applied to the skin and mu-cous membranes of the eye, vagina, anus and nose. Unlike creams, their lack of water means they have no need for preservatives, lessening the risk of ir-ritation and sensitization. Ointments are usually very moisturizing and therefore good for any con-dition characterized by dry skin. They are less eas-ily washed off than creams and, because they can also be messy, are less popular.

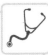

Clinical tip

An ointment may be better applied at night-time rather than during the day.

Gels

Gels have an active ingredient incorporated into a semi-solid hydrophilic (easily absorbed in water) or hydrophobic (incapable of dissolving in water) base. This contains a gelling agent, such as starch, making the base stiffer. Some of these can liquefy when they come into contact with warm skin.

Drying, so cooling, and not greasy, gels are particularly suited for applying to the face and scalp. Because of this drying effect, and perhaps also their alcoholic component, they may cause irritation, especially in acute lesions. Fluocinolone acetonide in gel formulation is often prescribed to treat scalp psoriasis. Clindomycin in gel formulation is used to treat facial acne.

Lotions

Although there is a significant variability in the basic ingredients of generic lotions when compared to brand name lotions, all are thin liquids. Composed mainly of a water base in which drugs can be dissipated or dispersed, they may contain alcohol. They can also be formulated as oil-in-water emulsions, and are used to treat dermatologic conditions, including acutely inflamed and weeping skin. As they spread easily and are not sticky, lotions are user-friendly when a large or hairy area of the body needs treating. The water or alcohol in the lotion formulation evaporates, giving a cooling sensation to the skin. Calamine lotion works in this way.

Clinical tip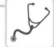

As with other aqueous preparations or those containing alcohol, lotions may cause irritation to raw areas or acute lesions. Their use may aggravate dryness of the skin. It is important to assess skin condition prior to application.

Lotions may be applied directly to the skin, or on swabs or dressings soaked in the lotion. In either case, frequent changing of dressings is necessary, otherwise the lotion will crust and cake. This may be avoided by the use of a liniment – a lotion with additional oil. This means dressings may be changed less frequently, but the cooling effect of rapid evaporation and its advantages are lost.

Pastes

These are stiff preparations (e.g. zinc paste) made by mixing powder into a grease base. They are useful for dry surfaces but can be difficult to remove.

Clinical tip

The following general rules are useful.

- Greasier ointments for dry, scaling skin.
- Watery creams for crusted, weeping lesions.
- Pastes where occlusion or longer action is needed.
- Gels for the face and scalp.
- Lotions for cooling and drying.

True topical medicines

This section addresses those preparations applied to the body surface (for external use only). In addition to true topical therapy, some conditions require the simultaneous use of oral drugs, or drugs administered via another route (e.g. injection). A huge variety of preparations is available for treating the body surface in both health and disease. Here we concentrate on the more common ones. Inevitably, some will be omitted.

Health and the treatment of common conditions

Maintaining a healthy skin is a priority. Caring for skin, hair and nails, our own, our children's, or that of people in our care is a concept we are brought up with and exposed to on a daily basis. The media constantly reminds us of what constitutes a 'beautiful' and 'youthful' skin and our need for it.

Changes in the skin can be intrinsic and specific to an individual or due to age and environmental factors. As well as treating skin disorders, infestations and a myriad of skin problems, true topical preparations are used to protect and keep the body surface healthy.

Sunscreens

Melanoma and skin cancers are more common in people experiencing prolonged over-exposure to the damaging ultraviolet B (UVB) rays of sunlight (UVA rays promote a tan). Sunburn in children, particularly under the age of 10, may increase this risk. Some conditions (e.g. herpes simplex) and some drugs can increase sensitivity to sunlight. This is also affected by skin type. The ageing effects of the sun on skin are well known.

On exposure to the UV rays of the sun, the melanocytes in the epidermis increase production of melanin. This, however, is an adaptive process – the skin may be damaged *before* adequate levels of melanin are produced. This necessitates avoiding exposure or applying screening agents before exposure. Chemicals in vehicles such as creams, oils and lotions contain agents which work in two different ways, absorbing the UV rays or reflecting them.

Absorbing sunscreens can be narrow or broad spectrum, depending on the wavelength they absorb. Those with a narrow spectrum (e.g. cinnamates, para-aminobenzoic acid and its esters) screen out UVB waves. These screening agents can stain and may cause photosensitivity. Broad spectrum screening agents (the benzophenones) are more efficient, screening out UVA and UVB rays. Opaque compounds such as zinc reflect the UV rays. Zinc oxide ointment is popular with surfers but less so with others as it is not very attractive cosmetically.

Whichever is chosen, all are formulated to remain on the skin surface, forming a physical barrier. This is important to remember. They should be applied frequently and according to instructions. Some are water resistant and will resist sweating; many are not, and are easily washed off when swimming. When buying a sunscreen its 'substantivity' is very important, as is considering the sun protective factor (SPF). This is a laboratory measure of the effectiveness of sunscreen – the higher the SPF, the more protection it offers against UVB rays. With an SPF of between 2 and 10, the sunscreen will be only mildly protective, rising to full protection with an SPF over 25. One word of caution: it has become a recent trend to put sunscreens with a very high SPF on children; however, this may prevent the synthesis of vitamin D, leading to a possible deficiency.

Deodorants and antiperspirants

While not thought of as medicines, the topical use of deodorants and antiperspirants to combat unpleasant body odour is commonplace. Every day, the human body produces an average of 1 litre of sweat. Typically, the apocrine glands release twice the amount of moisture as their eccrine counterparts. Given their location, it is less easy for the moisture produced by the apocrine glands to escape, and body odour may be more noticeable in these areas. Body odour is created as bacteria feed on the sweat produced by these glands (sweat itself has no smell). Washing will remove the micro-organisms and secretions which cause body odours, and perfumes can be used to mask them. Alternatively, the odour may be controlled by the topical use of either an antiperspirant or a deodorant.

Antiperspirants work by closing, clogging or blocking the pores that release perspiration, reducing moisture. They contain aluminium salts, which dissolve in the sweat, creating a thin coating of gel which covers the sweat glands, reducing the amount of sweat released onto the surface of the skin and giving bacteria less to feed on. Deodorants work differently – they do not stop perspiration but work by neutralizing the smell of perspiration by destroying the bacteria through the antimicrobials or alcohol contained within them. They will often contain a fragrance to mask the bad smells caused by the bacteria. Deodorants which inhibit the growth of micro-organisms commonly include chlorhexidine. Both deodorants and antiperspirants may be applied as a roll-on stick, a gel or a spray.

We have previously seen that the skin has an acid pH of 5.5 and this is important in protecting it against harmful bacteria. Continuous and excessive use of soap can increase the skin pH to 7.5. This increases the activity of the stratum corneum chymotryptic enzyme which can lead to a breakdown in the skin barrier, enabling allergens and irritants to enter the skin. Excessive washing

Dry Eczematous skin

Loss of moisture

Allergens penetrate the bricks and mortar

Not enough 'mortar'

Inflammation

Figure 8.4 Broken barrier in dry eczematous skin

not only removes dirt but also the skin's natural oils. Non-detergent neutral pH cleansers are available over the counter, and these may be preferable to harsh alkaline products.

Barrier creams

Nappy rash is commonly seen in babies, occuring when urine is broken down by bacteria, producing ammonia. This develops over time, but frequent changing of nappies will help prevent the problem. Applying barrier creams containing zinc oxide or silicone after bathing and at regular intervals will create a barrier between the urine and the skin, but in severe cases antibiotics and steroid creams may be necessary.

Dry skin

Dry skin is very common and can be caused by a variety of factors: the environment, excessive washing, poor diet, certain drugs, genetic factors, age and various skin conditions such as eczema, dermatitis and psoriasis. There is a lack of natural moisturizing factor in the keratinocytes and sebum from the oil glands, reducing the skin's lubrication and causing it to feel tight, flake, redden and, at worst, chap. This is caused by the 'mortar' breaking down between the corneocytes, causing them to dehydrate, shrink and crack (see Figure 8.4).

Dry skin may be graded as mild, moderate or severe. Once the skin's natural barrier is damaged it becomes open to attack from micro-organisms and allergens. When this happens, the skin's own inflammatory chemicals begin a counter-attack. This makes you itch, promoting scratching which

can further damage the skin. This creates the 'itch/scratch cycle' (see Figure 8.5).

Clinical tip

Under normal circumstances we experience an itch which, once scratched, disappears. Persistent, unrelenting and diffuse itchy skin is called *pruritis*, a distressing symptom affecting the physical integrity of the skin and the psychosocial well-being of a person. Pruritis can result in bleeding and scratching while asleep.

Emollients and moisturizers

Emollients and moisturizers are an essential and often underestimated treatment, significantly

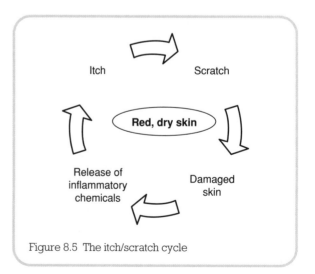

Itch

Scratch

Red, dry skin

Release of inflammatory chemicals

Damaged skin

Figure 8.5 The itch/scratch cycle

Effect of emollient and bath oil

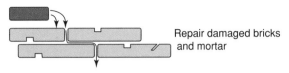

Repair damaged bricks and mortar

Emollients act like 'mortar' by filling in the gaps between the bricks (stratum corneum)

Figure 8.6 Effects of emollients on the stratum corneum

restoring dry skin and maintaining skin integrity. They may be used by themselves, without medication, making the skin not only feel but look better. All emollients contain *excipients*. With added active excipients, some products can reduce the symptoms of pruritis, inflammation and scaling.

> **Clinical tip**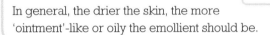
>
> In general, the drier the skin, the more 'ointment'-like or oily the emollient should be.

Although these terms are often used synonymously, there is a difference between an emollient and a moisturizer. Moisturizers are oily (lipid) emulsions containing *humectant* substances, often glycol or urea, that draw water towards them, actively adding moisture *to* the skin. Emollients are preparations which, used generously and frequently, prevent water loss *from* the skin. They do this passively, occluding the skin surface, thereby encouraging a build-up of water in the stratum corneum as well as penetrating the upper epithelial layers and repairing damaged 'mortar'.

Constituent ingredients in emollients vary. Most are oil based but some are oil free (useful for people with acne). They combine with a range of excipients to produce the vast array of emollient products on the market e.g. Aveeno, Diprobase and Oilatum to name but a few.

> **Clinical tip**
>
> Excipients in topical products rarely cause problems. Should they do so the product containing the substance should be avoided.

Emollients:

- Help with exfoliation.
- Have anti-inflammatory and anti-mitotic effects, especially if salicylic acid is added.
- Reduce itching through the addition of *lauromacrogols*. These are thought to reduce the transmission of itch sensations to the nerves. Anti-itch emollients are available as both leave-on and bathing products.
- Actively draw water up from the dermis into the epidermis if they contain humectants such as urea and glycol.

Some emollients contain both occlusive and humectant substances to maximize the hydrating effect, others contain benzalkonium chloride, chlorhexidine hydrochloride and triclosan which have an antiseptic effect. Emollients can be:

- Products left on the skin (ointments, creams, lotions).
- Washing products (bath additives and non-detergent skin cleansers). These can be added to the water and not rinsed off, leaving a thin layer of oil on the skin, preventing drying.
- A cleansing soap substitute which doesn't dry the skin and is rinsed off.

Using washing products alongside leave-on preparations will help reduce dry skin. Complete emollient therapy removes the need for soaps and detergents and incorporates the use of an emollient bath oil or shower gel, an emollient soap substitute for cleansing and a leave-on emollient applied liberally and frequently. Its effectiveness relies on an underlying knowledge and understanding of how emollients work.

Aqueous cream is an emollient with a high water content and should not be used as a leave-on product. Aqueous preparations were never intended to be left on the skin but are designed as a soap substitute. When left on the skin they can cause stinging and discomfort.

Clinical tip

Always ensure a product is used for the purpose for which it was designed. This may be especially true for over-the-counter products.

- Emollients may irritate the skin and cause contact dermatitis.
- Greasy emollients will make the bath slippery and precautions must be taken.
- There is a potential fire hazard if paraffin-based emollients are used in large quantities and come into contact with clothing which is then brought into close proximity with open and exposed fire sources.
- Occlusive ointments will inhibit heat loss and this may cause overheating.
- Warming emollients in winter may make them more comfortable and soothing; putting them in the fridge in summer helps to cool the skin and lessens the urge to scratch.

Frequent use of emollients, up to four times a day, would normally require 600g/week for an adult and 250g/week for a child. Pump dispensers containing large amounts of emollient are available. Two pumps per area such as the arm, thigh, shin, chest, abdomen, upper back and lower back are needed for light application, rising to five pumps for a medium-dose regime and more for a high dose determined by need.

Choosing an emollient

Choosing the appropriate type of emollient lotion, cream or ointment can be difficult. A golden rule

is that the greater proportion of oil, the more effective the preparation will be in keeping the skin hydrated. Choosing the correct emollient involves the consideration of several factors:

- an assessment of the nature and location of the problem;
- continence;
- age;
- lifestyle.

While it may be acceptable to use a greasy product in the bath or at night-time, a lighter cream may be more acceptable during the day. For very light use and to cool the skin, a lotion may be a better choice.

Clinical tip

Empowering patients to choose their own treatments is now well established practice. With support that ensures understanding, patients and their families can often self-manage the uncomplicated but persistent symptoms experienced in some skin disorders.

Infestations

Infestations are common and can include insect bites, parasitic infestations of the skin and hair and some less common tropical diseases beyond the scope of this chapter.

Insect repellents

Insect bites can be not only a nuisance but also fatal. Severe reactions require immediate medical help. Many over-the-counter preparations are available to counter the effect of insect bites including calamine lotion, antiseptic creams and alcohols.

Products are available in various vehicles (lotions, cream, sticks and sprays) and contain active ingredients including diethyl toluamide and dimethyl phthalate which, on vaporizing, repel insects. The more rapid the vaporization, the quicker the effect will wear off. This is also affected by washing and rubbing. The manufacturer's instructions for use must be followed carefully. While considered generally safe, diethyl toluamide and dimethyl phthalate can be absorbed and sensitization, which may become worse with prolonged use, can occur.

> **Clinical tip**
>
> A hot bath should be avoided after application of topical drugs, as an increase in skin temperature may increase absorption through the stratum corneum and into the blood.

Scabies

Scabies is a common worldwide skin disease caused by the small mite *Sarcoptes scabiei*. Gaining access to human skin through very close contact with an infected person, the female mite burrows into the stratum corneum, laying eggs en route. The male dies after completing his role of fertilization, and the developing eggs hatch into larvae under the skin, taking about two weeks to mature. Not surprisingly, this under-the-skin activity causes intense itching, however scabies can be easily missed or misdiagnosed. Characteristically, the distribution of the infestation is the fingers, wrists, abdomen, nipples, umbilicus, genitalia, buttocks and ankles. Infestation does not occur above the neck. Diagnosis can be difficult, because the affected area is often red and obscured through scratching. If uncertain, identification of mites or skin scrapings taken from a lesion will confirm the diagnosis. Treatments include permethrin, which is applied in a 0.5 per cent preparation thinly to the whole body, avoiding the eyes and broken skin. This application should be washed off after 8–12 hours and used twice, one week apart. Malathion is an alternative and is applied in a 0.5 per cent preparation in the same way as permethrin. Benzyl benzoate is a less effective preparation and also an irritant. It should not be used on children,

and the adult treatment involves the application of an emulsion over the whole body which is repeated after 24 hours. A third application may be necessary.

> **Clinical tip**
>
>
>
> A clean paintbrush is useful when applying the above. With the exception of benzyl benzoate, all family members should be treated, paying particular attention to the webs of the fingers and toes and brushing lotion under the ends of the fingers. Treatment must be reapplied if hands are washed within eight hours. Residual papules may persist for many weeks.

Anti-inflammatory creams and topical steroids can be used to relieve the itching, and secondary infection as a result of scratching may need to be treated. Itching may persist even after all the mites have been eliminated; papules on the scrotum and penis are particularly persistent. Children with scabies should be excluded from school until 24 hours after treatment

If scabies does not respond to topical treatment alone it can be combined with a single dose of the oral drug ivermectin.

Burrowed mites do not survive in bedding and cannot be transmitted by clothing or lavatory seats. The body, however, does not acquire immunity to scabies infestation and treatment does not prevent another attack.

Hair

Under normal circumstances appropriate washing and hair brushing will keep the head hair and scalp healthy, removing dirt, grease and dead keratinocytes. To aid this process there are shampoos and hair conditioning products available for all ages, hair types and preferences. An increase in the normal production and shedding of keratinocytes from the scalp is called dandruff, an itchy but harmless condition varying in severity. Persistent or excessive dandruff is associated with an inflammation of the scalp called *seborrhoeic dermatitis*. Often caused by a yeast, a rash along the hairline may be present in severe cases. This can be treated with the regular use of shampoos medicated with zinc pyrithione or selenium sulphide, or those containing coal tar or salicylic acid. These latter preparations reduce the overproduction of new skin cells and break down the keratin in the excessive cells (keratolytic agents) which are then washed off. Ointments of coal tar are also available. Severe seborrhoeic dermatitis can be treated with an antifungal shampoo containing ketoconazole. This reduces the overgrowth of yeast on the scalp. Corticosteroid gels and lotions may relieve a very itchy rash on the scalp.

Hair loss can be due to alopecia (which can be caused by ringworm), psoriasis, disorders of the follicles themselves or as a response to illness. Other factors may be malnutrition or the use of anti-cancer drugs or anticoagulants. Each cause should be treated on an individual basis. Normal male pattern hair loss (*androgenic alopecia*) can be treated with topical minoxidil as well as oral finasteride.

The hair on our heads, bodies and pubic region can also become infested with lice if allowed to come into direct contact with them.

Lice

Infestation with head lice (*pediculosis capitis*) is common. Spread by close head-to-head contact, lice move from the hair of one infected person to that of another. They can be found in all types and lengths of hair. Having head lice is not a sign that hair is dirty, they are just as often found living in clean hair. Head lice are particularly common among children (aged 4–11 especially) because they tend to have more head-to-head contact at school or during play, but they can affect anyone with hair. Head lice cannot fly, jump or swim, nor infest furniture, bedding or pets. They must have a human host and will die without one. They live on the scalp, preferring the back of the head and above and behind the ears, where it is warmer.

Although people with head lice may not have any symptoms, itching (particularly behind the ears

and the nape of the neck) is common. Observing children scratching their head may be an indicator. Excessive scratching may cause the skin to become broken and infections can develop. Diagnosis is made by directly observing a louse or nit, or through detection by combing wet hair (this immobilizes the louse) using a specially designed head lice comb. You should also check for white shiny empty shells (nits). These remain cemented to the hair after the lice have hatched and can be mistaken for flakes of skin or dandruff. They stick to the hairs as they grow out and cannot be washed off with normal shampoo, needing physical removal from the hair.

Head lice will not go away on their own. They need treatment, usually with topical pediculicides (insecticides) which kill them and their eggs. Medicated lotions can be prescribed or bought over the counter, and are effective provided the manufacturer's instructions are followed. Evidence of resistance to preparations continues to increase, however, and head lice repellents are no longer considered effective.

Lice can also be removed by wet combing ('bug busting') and there are some non-insecticidal products available over the counter.

Clinical tip

If you suspect head lice, or that an individual has been in contact with someone with confirmed head lice, it is important to check all contacts, ensuring all cases can be treated simultaneously.

Various forms of treatment are available. Dimethicone lotion (4 per cent) is not an insecticide and acts effectively, coating the surface of the organism, affecting its breathing and distorting water balance. Colourless, it has no smell and a slightly oily consistency. It should be applied to all of the hair, and left to dry naturally, washing out eight hours later. As with insecticides, the treatment will need to be reapplied after seven days to kill any new lice that have hatched. Dimethicone does not irritate the scalp, and lice cannot become resistant to it.

Malathion (Derbac) 0.5 per cent is an insecticide useful for all types of louse infestation. At least two applications of the product, seven days apart, are needed, ensuring that any lice hatching after the first treatment are killed. A maximum of three treatments should be used in any one course.

Isopropyl myristate 50 per cent in cyclomethicone solution ('Full Marks' solution) is a non-insecticide oily liquid which has to be combed through the hair and washed off after 10 minutes. Full Marks solution soaks into the louse's coat and appears to block its breathing tubes.

These products are either alcohol-based or water-based, and there does not seem to be any difference in effectiveness between the two. Alcohol-based insecticides are not suitable for everyone, particularly those with eczema or asthma. Water-based products are usually recommended in such cases. These products are also recommended for young children, but not those aged under 2, when the use of wet combing (see below) is preferable.

The patient should always be reminded to follow any instructions carefully, noting special considerations for pregnancy and breastfeeding. The lotion should usually be rubbed onto the scalp and hair and left for at least 12 hours before washing out. Shampoos and foams are not recommended, as they do not remain in contact with the lice long enough to kill them.

Finally, remember that some insecticides can cause side-effects, including scalp irritation and eczema. The patient and family should be informed that repeated treatments with insecticides are not recommended without further advice from a health professional e.g. doctor or pharmacist. These products should only be used if there is a head lice infestation, never as a precaution.

A follow-up check should be carried out a few days after completing the course. Finding eggs does not necessarily mean that the treatment has failed. The lice may have been killed and these could be empty egg cases. If a live adult louse is found, it may be because the person has become reinfested.

Wet combing

This procedure does not involve chemicals, and lice cannot become resistant to it. It can also be used for routinely checking the hair for infection. Using a comb designed for very fine combing (a nit comb), every section of wet hair needs to be carefully combed (remembering to protect your own hair), removing lice. Repeatedly going over the head, this process should take about half an hour.

Other types of lice

It is possible for people to have body lice (*pediculosis corporis*) and/or pubic lice (*pediculosis pubis*). Those with body lice may present with itching, scratch marks and secondary infections. The seams of clothing should be examined because this is where lice may be found. If infestation is confirmed, all clothing should be removed and fumigated with malathion or an alternative parasiticide. The body requires one treatment of 0.5 per cent malathion. Topical steroids may also be needed to relieve symptoms.

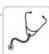

> **Clinical tip**
>
> If a person presents with body lice, it is always good practice to check for head lice and scabies.

Pubic lice are transmitted through close body contact, and cause itching. Having sucked blood from the area, the lice appear as blue black 'dots' in the pubic hair. Sexual partners should be treated at the same time.

Warts

These are localized areas of hyperkeratinization caused by the human papilloma virus. This virus may infect the skin for a long time before the body realizes it is present and starts to mount an attack. Warts most commonly occur on the hands and soles of the feet. Also called 'plantar warts' or 'verrucas', these may be painful due to pressure from shoes and cause local damage. Warts can also occur on the face and anogenital areas, requiring medical treatment.

Treatment

There is no ideal treatment for warts. Products available include paints, ointments, gels, plasters and treatment kits. Most of these products contain salicylic acid, a long-standing remedy which weakens the cement material (mortar) in the stratum corneum, stimulating its shedding, along with the wart. With careful attention and detailed application, wart paint will generally remove a wart. Other treatments are available. Silver nitrate may be applied, either from a toughened pencil or as a solution onto the lesion. This treatment produces a black *eschar* (piece of dead tissue), which eventually drops off. Formaldehyde and gluteraldehyde are believed to be antiviral and are also effective. These have a drying effect. Soaking in warm water for a few minutes prior to treatment may help penetration and enhance activity. Formaldehyde soaks are good for treating multiple warts in the same area. Left untreated, warts will eventually clear up on their own.

Clinical tip

Salicylic acid will damage both healthy and damaged keratin. Healthy skin around the wart should be protected with soft paraffin. Wart plasters are helpful in treating the infected area and also protect healthy surrounding skin.
If a wart looks suspicious, or is particularly dark and bleeding, a patient should seek medical advice. Remember that in patients undergoing cytotoxic therapy or those who are immunosuppressed, proliferation may be uncontrollable.

Skin disorders

Skin problems are very common and frequently very debilitating. It is estimated that about 25 per cent of the UK population has a skin disorder and 19 per cent of these will consult their doctor. Caring for patients with a dermatological condition, therefore, represents a significant workload for health professionals. As a student, it is highly likely that you will come across an individual with a skin complaint.

The three main chronic relapsing skin conditions (psoriasis, eczema and acne) each need an individual approach as no two patients are the same. Seeking a cure is not a viable outcome in chronic relapsing skin disorders such as psoriasis or eczema. Quite often, the most difficult problem for the patient is learning to live with the condition.

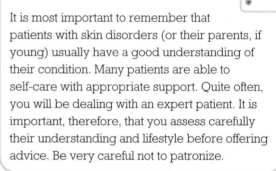

Clinical tip

It is most important to remember that patients with skin disorders (or their parents, if young) usually have a good understanding of their condition. Many patients are able to self-care with appropriate support. Quite often, you will be dealing with an expert patient. It is important, therefore, that you assess carefully their understanding and lifestyle before offering advice. Be very careful not to patronize.

The majority of medication used in dermatology is applied topically and such drugs are the first line of treatment in chronic skin disorders such as eczema and psoriasis.

Eczema

The term 'eczema', often used interchangeably with 'dermatitis', refers to a set of symptoms and a pattern of inflammatory responses in the skin. It should not be thought of as a disease, and is most definitely not contagious. 'Eczema' and 'dermatitis' are now used interchangeably, although 'dermatitis' was previously used to imply an occupational cause. Several different types of eczema are known, and are generally classified as either:

- exogenous (from the outside); or
- endogenous (from within, or atopic).

Often referred to as *contact dermatitis*, the exogenous type results from allergens or irritants. The endogenous form is also known as *constitutional* and *atopic* and has further classifications. The term 'atopic' is used where there is a a hereditary or constitutional tendency to develop hypersensitivity reactions. Eczma may also take a multi-factorial form, combining both of the above. It may be acute, sub-acute, infected and chronic. Because of its wide variety of clinical features and the terms applied, it can be a confusing disorder. In addition, a patient with one form of eczema may well develop another.

Characteristics and features

The common identifying characteristics of the four types are:

- **Acute:** red (erythema) abnormally dry skin, vesicles and blisters.
- **Sub-acute:** erythema, exudates, crusts, scaling and excoriation.
- **Infected:** weeping, oozing, crusting and pustulation.
- **Chronic:** dry, scaly skin with fissures and lichenification (thickening of the skin).

These may not all appear together, and can be of varying severity. All are a result of inflammatory changes giving rise to the characteristic symptoms of itching (pruritis), redness and heat. We have already discussed the problem of itchy skin and this is most troublesome in eczema, where there may be a low threshold for itching. The itch/scratch cycle becomes an important feature, causing misery for the sufferer. Children in particular can become very irritable because of constant itching and sleepless nights. They may be teased and stigmatized at school, making them even more miserable and affecting their concentration.

A number of factors can trigger an acute form of eczema or make the condition worse, especially agents that dry skin further or increase the urge to scratch. Hormonal factors such as the menstrual cycle and pregnancy have been identified as affecting the symptoms. Much of the true topical treatment is aimed at reducing itching which, if left unchecked, leads to excoriation and lichenification due to excessive rubbing and possible infection.

Exogenous eczema

This may be due to contact with common allergens which promote an allergic response. Examples include nickel, chromate, perfume, lanolin, preservatives found in cosmetics and shampoos, harsh detergents and soap, oils and solvents. Earlier in this chapter we discussed excipients (additives). Exposure to these may also cause contact dermatitis. Avoidance, both at home and at work, of allergens known to cause sensitivity is important.

Endogenous (atopic) eczema

Examples include:

- **Seborrhoeic:** affecting the scalp. It is called 'cradle cap' in babies and dandruff in adults, and may also affect the face and ear canal.
- **Discoid:** causing disc-shaped lesions primarily on the limbs.
- **Gravitational:** associated with impaired venous drainage.
- **Pompholyx:** blistering of the hands and feet.
- **Asteatotic:** excessive dryness of the skin.

The prevalence of atopic eczema is increasing. It is a chronic inflammatory disorder with a genetic component and the culprit is believed to be an inherited defective gene (or genes) in the skin's immune system. Although not fully understood, it is believed that this results in a reduced cellular responsiveness to microbial antigens and heightened antibody responses. Atopic eczema is associated with asthma and hay fever. Skin inflammation caused by allergens or irritants provokes the mast and white defensive blood cells to release substances that dilate the local blood vessels, making the skin red, hot and swollen.

Infection is said to be the 'hidden dimension' of eczema. The skin of patients with atopic eczema has high levels of a bacterium called *Staphylococcus aureus*, correlating with the severity of the eczema. When combined with environmental factors, this triggers an overreaction of antibodies. An absence or reduction of the protein filaggrin is found in those suffering from eczema. This leads to drying of the skin, poor barrier function in the outer skin and excessive peeling away or *desquamation* of dead, dry skin. The 'mortar' between the keratinocytes in the stratum corneum becomes defective and the barrier function is impaired, making the skin very dry and the cells irregular in shape. This allows bacteria to stick to them and, as we have seen, a defective barrier makes the skin both dry and vulnerable to penetration by irritants and allergens. Eczema often begins in infancy and has a family history.

The orthodox approach to treatment

Eczema is not a disease but a set of symptoms. It cannot be cured but the aim is to control the symptoms through:

- accurate assessment and diagnosis;
- identification and removal of causative factors where possible;
- alleviation of dryness and itchiness;
- recognition and treatment of any secondary infection;
- teamwork, education and patient involvement and choice, maximizing concordance.

Eczema responds to topical therapy which may involve the following.

- Total emollient therapy. The mainstay of treatment, this prevents dry skin and cracking.
- Using alternatives to soap.
- Applying topical corticosteroids of an appropriate strength in an appropriate vehicle to the site.
- Eliminating inflammation as a result of infection through the use of an antibiotic cream with a low sensitizing potential.
- Use of paste bandages containing zinc or Ichthammol for the more lichenified and chronically dry types of eczema. These bandages are antipruritic, soothing and hydrating. They may be applied over a corticosteroid.

- The use of systemic antihistamines and antibiotics.
- Wet/dry wraps.

Wet/dry wrap therapy

Wet wrapping involves the application of liberal amounts of emollient under garments specifically designed for the purpose. Current practice uses tubular garments such as vests, leggings, shorts and gloves in different sizes. For dry wrapping the garment is put on over the emollient. In wet wrapping the garment is warmed in a bowl of water (approximately the temperature of washing-up water) prior to wringing out and applying to the body over the emollient or primary dressing such as a zinc paste bandage if the eczema is severe. A dry garment is then added. Wet wraps can be used throughout the day in the right conditions as long as hydration is maintained by frequent damping/spraying of the lower layer and the climate is controlled.

Clinical tip

Wet wrapping must not be used if there are any obvious signs of infection.

The potenital benefits of this type of therapy are:

- skin rehydration;
- more restful sleep;
- reduced redness and inflammation;
- less frequent itching;
- the emollient is prevented from being wiped off and clothing is protected;
- a wet garment helps to increase the penetration of prescribed topical treatments.

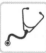

Clinical tip

The best time to wet wrap is just after a bath. An emollient could be used in the bath for dry itchy skin instead of soap.

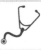

Use of emollients

Given that a characteristic of eczema is dry skin, the use of emollients is particularly important in its treatment.

- Most people with eczema have associated dry skin requiring emollient use. This may be underestimated in both the need and the frequency to achieve maximum effect.
- Continual use of complete emollient therapy will help provide maximum relief.
- The use of emollients far outweighs other therapies and should exceed corticosteroid use by 10:1 in terms of quantity. This in turn will reduce the need for topical corticosteroids.
- Using an emollient with added lauromacrogols (surfactant) should help to break the itch/scratch cycle.

Use of topical steriods

Steroids have been used in dermatology to relieve itching and suppress inflammation since 1952 and remain in common use for a variety of skin disorders, including psoriasis, eczema and other types of dermatitis. Preparations include ointments, creams and lotions. They are effective and safe when used appropriately although many people feel cautious about their use. Topical steroids are available in four strengths or potencies: mild, moderate, potent and very potent. Some examples are given below.

- **Mild:** hydrocortisone 0.1–2.5 per cent. In general, mild corticosteroids can be safely given to treat acute inflammatory skin lesions of the face and flexural areas.
- **Moderate:** alclometasone, clobetasone and fluocortolone. Flurandrenalones are often required to treat chronic, hyperkeratotic or lichenified lesions on the palms or soles.
- **Potent:** beclomethasone, betamethasone, desoxymethasone, diflucortolone, fluocinolone, fluocinonide, fluticasone, mometasone, triamcinolone.
- **Very potent:** clobetasol, halcinonide.

> **Clinical tip**
>
> Skin creams and ointments containing hydrocortisone can be bought over the counter for the treatment of insect bites and mild to moderate eczema.

Different dermatology teams may use different regimens but topical steroid preparations should be applied no more frequently than twice daily, and once daily is often sufficient. In most cases corticosteroid treatment is begun with a low dose. The aim is to get the best result with the least potent medicine although a stronger preparation may be required.

> **Clinical tip**
>
> The more inflamed and active the atopic eczema the greater the potential for absorption of the drug into the bloodstream through the damaged stratum corneum.

Topical steroids are contraindicated in untreated bacterial, fungal or viral skin lesions. Side-effects can be associated with mild and moderately potent steroids. These include:

- spread and worsening of untreated infections;
- thinning of the skin, which may be restored to a certain extent once treatment stops;
- irreversible striae atrophicae and telangiectasia;
- contact dermatitis;
- acne or worsening of acne or rosacea.

Topical steroids are spread thinly on the skin. The length of cream or ointment expelled from a tube may be used to specify the quantitiy to be applied to a given area of skin, measured in terms of a 'fingertip unit' – the distance from the tip of the adult index finger to the first crease. This equates with approximately 0.5g.

The quantities for prescribing on specific areas of the body are listed below. These amounts are usually suitable for an adult for a single daily application for a two week period.

- Face and neck 15–30g
- Both hands 15–30g
- Scalp 15–30g
- Both arms 30–60g
- Both legs 100g
- Trunk 100g
- Groin and genitalia 15–30g

Tacrolimus ointment

This is an *immunomodulatory* drug (it changes the immune system), *not* a steroid, available on prescription only. It is used for the treatment of moderate to very severe eczema that is unresponsive to conventional therapy. Available in two different strengths it is applied thinly to the skin twice a day. It must be used with plenty of emollient but is not suitable for use under wet wraps. It may cause a burning sensation and sun exposure should be limited when undergoing treatment. It is also used for psoriasis.

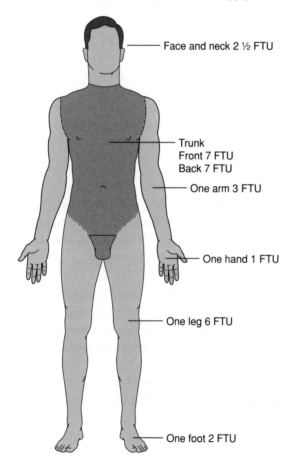

Guidelines on the amount of eczema cream to apply in adults

1 FTU = 1/2 gramme
2 FTU = 1 gramme

Face and neck 2 ½ FTU

Trunk
Front 7 FTU
Back 7 FTU

One arm 3 FTU

One hand 1 FTU

One leg 6 FTU

One foot 2 FTU

= 1 FTU

Guidelines in children
Face and neck, arm and hand, leg and foot, trunk (front), trunk (back and buttock)

Figure 8.7 Guidelines for application of finger tip units

- Widespread small plaque
- Guttate psoriasis
- Facial psoriasis
- Flexural psoriasis
- Pustular psoriasis
- Acute erythrodermis
- Unstable or generalized pustular psoriasis

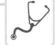

Clinical tip

There are national guidelines for a stepped care plan for managing atopic eczema in children (see NICE 2008).

Psoriasis

Psoriasis is one of the common skin disorders said to affect about 2 per cent of the population. Occurring equally in men and women of any age, its onset is usually in early adult life. In psoriasis sufferers the rate of orthokeratosis (renewal of the skin) is dramatically increased. There is increased thickness of the epidermis, presence of nuclei above the basal layer and thicker than normal keratin in the 'bricks' of the stratum corneum. Although the exact cause of psoriasis is not known there is evidence that hormonal and immunological mechanisms are involved at a cellular level and it is believed there is a genetic component also. The disorder is characterized by epidermal thickening and scaling.

Because the epidermis is dividing so rapidly, the cells in each layer do not have time to develop in the normal way. The keratinocytes in the stratum corneum resemble a faulty brick wall – built too high in too much of a hurry it becomes structurally unsound, with the 'tumbling bricks' representing the scales. The redness (erythema) is due to the nearby dilated blood vessels. There are equivalent changes in the nails, causing thickening and pitting.

Several factors may induce the onset of an episode of psoriasis, including stress or a throat infection (especially true of children). Patches of psoriasis (also called *plaques*) are pink or red, have a well-defined edge and are covered by thick, silvery-white scales. They occur mainly on the knees, elbows, trunk or scalp, although any area can be affected. Although unsightly the disorder is not infectious but is frequently itchy.

Psoriasis can take several forms which affect various parts of the body:

- Stable plaque
- Extensive stable plaque

Psoriasis can be drug-induced – examples include lithium, NSAIDs and angiotensin-converting enzyme (ACE) inhibitors.

Treatment

Treatment is conducted with ointments and pastes, oral systemic drugs and various forms of UV light. Treatment is tailored to the type of psoriasis, the patient's age, lifestyle and personal preference, aiding concordance. Creams and ointments applied to the areas of psoriasis are medically prescribed. Sunlight usually improves the condition, although it has been known to make it worse. Diet is not thought to have any effect. A positive attitude which expects improvement (but not permanent cure) is essential. Emollients are used to treat dry skin and to prevent skin cracking and scaling. These may also have an anti-proliferative effect. More specific treatments include the use of vitamin D analogues, dithranol, coal tar and the retinoid tartrazine.

The use of dithranol and coal tars has taken a 'back seat' in modern dermatology; vitamin D analogues are clean and odourless and can be very effective. They include calcipotriol, calcitriol and tacalcitol.

Calcipotriol

Calcipotriol is a man-made form of vitamin D and is the first-line treatment for mild to moderate plaque psoriasis. It is thought to slow down the rate of skin cell division and reduce skin inflammation. It may be combined with other topical agents or with phototherapy. Using calcipotriol and topical corticosteroids together produces fewer side-effects than treating with either agent alone. Knowledge of how different topical medicines interact with calcipotriol is required when it is used in combination therapy as several topical medicines, including salicylic acid, inactivate calcipotriol.

Clinical tip

Calcipotriol is not the same as the vitamin D bought in a chemists or health-food shops. This has no value in treating psoriasis.

The advantages of this medicine are that it can be used in areas where corticosteroids may not be recommended, including the eyelids and areas where skin folds occur. The patient also benefits from having relatively long periods of remission when the drug is used alongside a steroid. Cosmetically acceptable to individuals, its side-effects are relatively mild. The disadvantages include the usual suspects such as skin irritation. It should be used with care in young children, as it can affect bone growth.

Dithranol

This medicine belongs to a group of agents called the *anthroquinilones* which slow down keratinocyte division (an antimitotic effect). Any one of a number of brands can be prescribed for home use. Dithranol can be used in a paste containing salicylic acid, zinc oxide, starch and soft white paraffin. Other preparations and concentrations are available. An ointment may be more effective but (as with all vehicles) the water-washable creams may be more cosmetically acceptable. It can be used as either short- or long-term contact therapy. As it is a skin irritant, areas of thinner skin with a high absorption capacity should be avoided. It should not be used in active lesions and application to normal skin should also be avoided. Dithranol should not be applied to the bends (flexures) of the elbows or knees without medical advice as this will encourage irritation in these areas.

Clinical tip

It is important to protect the healthy skin around lesions by using a petroleum-based vehicle.

Short contact therapy using dithranol means applying the cream and leaving it on for a short time before washing off. Treatment is usually carried out once a day. Avoiding contact with the eyes, dithranol should be applied sparingly and rubbed gently (only onto the affected areas) until the cream is absorbed. Remember to remind the patient to wash their hands following application. Between half an hour and an hour later the cream should be removed by bathing or showering (using soap or shower gel). The patient should apply an emollient immediately and clean the bath or shower with a proprietary cleanser to avoid permanent staining. Dithranol stains clothes, so old clothes should be worn until the cream is washed off.

As the psoriasis begins to clear, the treated areas will gradually stain brown. The strength of the dithranol used is gradually increased every three to five days from 0.1 per cent to a maximum strength of 2 per cent. If treated areas become inflamed, treatment should cease until this settles. Once this happens, treatment can begin again at a lower concentration. When the psoriasis clears, treatment ceases. This can, however, take a number of weeks. The staining will disappear in a couple of weeks. If new plaques return, they can be re-treated with dithranol in the same way.

If psoriasis does not respond to short-contact dithranol therapy or is too severe for home management, long-contact therapy may be needed which requires medical management, either as an inpatient or, more frequently, as an outpatient.

Topical steroids

Steroids may be used under close supervision, but the same rules apply to their use in treating psoriasis as they do for other topical applications. The weaker steroids may not work very well for thicker patches of psoriasis. There is also a tendency for psoriasis to be suppressed by topical steroids, but to rebound quickly when treatment stops. Mild steroid creams can be used on the scalp, hands and feet.

Tar preparations

Coal tar is effective for chronic plaque psoriasis. It can be incorporated into various vehicles, often pastes, which remain on the skin longer, having a longer effect. Tar products work in a similar way to dithranol, but are less of an irritant. Standard coal tar pastes are safe and effective for stable plaque-type psoriasis but are difficult to use at home. They smell, stain, are messy and will irritate acute inflamed areas. Numerous proprietary preparations are available in cream, ointment, gel and lotion forms. Some preparations contain salicylic acid and an emollient to aid keratolysis in thick scaly lesions. Others come with added hydrocortisone such as Alphosyl HC and Carbo-Cort. Refined coal tar extracts can be used for less severe areas of psoriasis. Tar preparations in the form of a shampoo are especially useful for use on the scalp (e.g. Polytar, Capasal and Slphosyl).

In severe psoriasis, coal tar may be combined with UV light therapy. This combination therapy, known as the Goeckerman treatment, has been shown to clear psoriasis in many patients in about three to four weeks. To receive treatment, patients must attend specialized centres for daily therapy.

Icthammol

This medicine, prepared from shale rather than coal tar, is less irritating and more soothing for inflamed skin. It is better for unstable or inflamed psoriasis when tar would not be tolerated. It can be made up as 1 per cent in yellow soft paraffin with 15 per cent zinc oxide.

> **Clinical tip**
>
> The British Association of Dermatology advocates *rotational therapy*, whereby topical treatments are alternated. This helps to lessen the likelihood of intolerance.

Retinoids

Retinoids belong to a group of drugs derived from vitamin A (found in yellow fruit and vegetables) and act on the skin to cause drying and peeling and a reduction in oil. They can be used in the treatment of acne, psoriasis and other skin disorders. Retinoids normalize DNA activity in skin cells, which decreases their rapid growth. Retinoids include tretinoin and isotretinoin.

Tazarotene is a man-made retinoid approved for the treatment of mild to moderate plaque psoriasis. It has also been reported to be effective in treating psoriasis of the nails. Available by prescription only, tazarotene comes in cream and gel forms. Local skin irritation is a common side-effect. When used in combination with topical corticosteroids, the effects of tazarotene are enhanced, skin irritation is decreased and some of the side-effects from the corticosteroids are reduced. Tazarotene is not recommended for use in areas where skin folds occur due to possible skin irritation. Although the possibility of birth defects is much lower for topical retinoids than for the systemic forms, women who are pregnant, or who may become pregnant, should use topical retinoids only under close medical supervision.

Pimecrolimus and tacrolimus

These are new drugs used to treat psoriasis. Both pimecrolimus and tacrolimus are topical immunomodulators. When applied to the skin, they exert a powerful anti-inflammatory effect. Tacrolimus can be safely applied to the eyelids and other areas around the eye, where topical corticosteroids must be used with caution. Side-effects are the same as for eczema. Treatment can be completely effective but, as with all treatments, even if the psoriasis disappears there is a tendency for it to return.

Acne

Many of us will have experienced spots, particularly on the face, when we were growing up. More troublesome and persistent spots are referred to as acne. *Acne vulgaris* (common acne) is believed to affect 15 per cent of adolescents. Without effective treatment it can reach its peak between the ages of 17 and 21. Most people become spot free by the age of 25; however, acne may persist well beyond adulthood and can affect people aged 40 and over. It may even begin in adulthood, brought on by environmental conditions or industrial chemicals.

Although acne may be mild and harmless, its psychological effects cannot be underestimated. Spots may develop into lesions which can rupture and cause deep dermal inflammation leading to scarring in the long term.

Altered physiology

Acne is an inflammatory condition in which there is increased production of sebum from the pilosebaceous units in the skin (sebaceous glands and their ducts) resulting in the hair follicles becoming blocked. Since these glands occur mainly on the face, neck, back and chest, these are the main sites affected by acne. The sebaceous glands are under the influence of the sex hormones, which is why acne commonly occurs at puberty and affects both sexes. It is not associated with an increase in hormones but more with an over-response to them by the sebaceous glands. The excessive production of sebum is also associated with hyperkeratosis and a blockage of the pilosebaceous duct, allowing the *Propionibacterium* acne organisms to multiply. This can result in a release of inflammatory cytokines resulting in turn in inflammation around the sebaceous gland, causing lesions.

Clinical features

People with acne will often be aware of, and concerned about, the increased oiliness of their skin. They will also notice that not all the spots are the same. Most people recognize a blackhead or *comedome* (which is the medical term), one feature of acne. Open comedomes are plugs of keratin which contain melanin and block the opening of the sebaceous duct; closed comedomes (whiteheads) are small white or skin-coloured spots. These often outnumber the open comedomes. Comedomes can develop into more inflamed lesions – small red lumps called *papules*, and yellow pus-filled spots called *pustules*.

Spots may become tender and more inflamed, creating the larger nodules and cysts. These may lead to scarring of the skin. If scars do form, they may be small depressions in the skin (atrophic scars) or raised from its surface (keloid scars). Irritant substances may gain access to the damaged

skin barrier. The spots occurring on black skin can become much darker and this can last a long time, even months.

Clinical tip

Although acne may be considered a relatively harmless disorder, it can have a devastating effect, both physically and psychologically, so active early treatment, education and management are important. The patient should be advised to avoid picking the lesions. While it is a myth that dirty people get acne, sufferers should wash the affected areas regularly to reduce greasiness. Over-the-counter antibacterial lotions and soaps may be of limited use, possibly drying the skin and causing irritation. Moderate exposure to sunlight may help.

Treatment

Management strategies relate to the severity and pathology of acne, incorporating several true topical medicines which work in different ways. Some preparations can be bought over the counter, others need a prescription. Treatments include anticomedonal agents, topical antimicrobials, retinoids and occasionally anti-androgen preparations. Steroids should not be used in treating acne.

Moderate to severe acne needs early and sustained treatment to prevent scarring and control exacerbation. Mild to moderate acne generally responds to true topical treatment although moderate to severe conditions may require oral medication in the form of antibiotics.

Anticomedonal (keratolytic) skin preparations encourage the dead cells of the stratum corneum to peel off. This helps unblock the pilosebaceous hair follicles and clear the comedomes, allowing the sebum to flow freely. Examples include benzoyl peroxide and salicylic acid. Available as creams, these have a keratolytic effect, eradicating *Propionibacterium* acne organisms. Benzoyl peroxide also has an antibacterial effect. The effect is often noticeable within a few weeks but it may take six weeks or longer before the acne improves. Some people have reported a flare up in their acne in the first few weeks of treatment which usually settles with continued use.

Adapalene is available as a cream and gel 0.1 per cent and is useful for mild to moderate acne. It is a retinoid-like drug and is less of an irritant than other topical retinoids. It is applied thinly before bedtime.

Topical naphthoic acid and derivatives are recommended for comedonal acne. They can also be used as monotherapy for uncomplicated acne. They are most often blended with antimicrobials as a combination therapy.

Topical antibiotics reduce bacteria and may also have a direct anti-inflammatory effect on the skin. They are *suppressive* not *curative* and are thought to affect the lipase-producing bacteria present in pilosebaceous follicles, countering bacterial activity. Antibacterial agents help to control the colonization of *Propionibacterium* acne organisms. Tetracycline is the first choice in treating acne. Examples of second-line antibiotics are erythromycin and trimethoprim. Topical antibiotics should be taken continuously for six months or even longer.

Finally, an option for acne treatment is to use agents which block the androgen receptor, thus blocking the effect of androgens on the sebaceous glands. A newer concept is the blocking of the activity of the androgen-metabolizing enzymes in the skin or in the sebaceous glands themselves. Such agents are called *anti-androgens*. The more common types in use are inocoterone acetate, spironolactone, cyproterone acetate, flutamide and the newer 5-alpha reductase inhibitors.

Clinical tip

Keratolytic agents often cause the skin at the site of treatment to be sore. If this persists, suggest that changing to a milder preparation may be beneficial.

Case studies

① Philip is 12 years old. He has had eczema since the age of 3 months. His eczema is normally kept under control with Aveeno cream applied daily. He hasn't needed any treatment other than emollients for two months. He has just come back from Scout camp (evening), where he was too embarrassed to be seen putting 'cream on' and had a flare-up of symptoms. He has generalized areas of dry, itchy and red excoriated skin and is not sleeping as a result. His eczema does not appear to be infected.

- What treatment does Philip need?
- Should he keep using his emollient?
- What additional treatments would be useful?

② You are a practice nurse working in an ethnic minority area. A young Muslim man, Bilal, who is a political asylum-seeker, comes to the clinic but doesn't speak English. You know from an interpreter that he has 'itchy skin' but he cannot explain the problem. You notice he is incessantly scratching his hands between his second and third fingers.

- What skin problem would this immediately alert you to?
- What treatment would you recommend?
- What advice would you give the patient via the interpreter?

Key learning points

Introduction

➤ The concept of 'topical' medicines and the topical route is complex.
➤ Many preparations applied to the skin or mucous membranes are not 'true topical'. They are designed to behave very differently, as they do not treat directly the part to which they have been applied.

Factors affecting the skin barrier

➤ An intact skin is essential. Non-intact skin has implications for the use of true topical preparations.

Drug absorption and the body surface

➤ Any medication applied to the body surface, whether for local or for systemic purposes, must be incorporated into an appropriate vehicle or base.

Occlusion

➤ The absorption of some drugs can be enhanced (10 to 100 times) through occlusion – the use of closed, airtight dressings or greasy ointment bases which increase hydration and the temperature of the stratum corneum.

Vehicles used to deliver drugs to the surface of the body

➤ Skin preparations make use of many different vehicle types: liquids, greases and powders mixed in various combinations to produce creams, ointments, lotions, gels and pastes.

Creams and ointments

➤ Considered as separate vehicles, creams or ointments may be used on their own, as emollients or as vehicles for active ingredients such as steroids and antimicrobials.

True topical medicines

➤ As well as treating skin disorders, infestations and a myriad of skin problems, true topical preparations are used to protect and keep the body surface healthy.

Dry skin

➤ Emollients and moisturizers are an essential and often underestimated treatment, significantly restoring dry skin and maintaining skin integrity.

Scabies

➢ Scabies is a common worldwide skin disease caused by the small mite *Sarcoptes scabiei*. Treatments included permethrin and malathion.

➢ All family members should be treated at the same time, paying particular attention to the webs of the fingers and toes.

Lice

➢ Infestation with head lice is common. It is spread by close head-to-head contact.

Warts

➢ There is no ideal treatment for warts. Products available include paints, ointments, gels, plasters and treatment kits. Most of these products contain salicylic acid.

Eczema

➢ The term 'eczema', often used interchangeably with 'dermatitis', refers to a set of symptoms and pattern of inflammatory responses in the skin. Exogenous eczema results from allergens or irritants. Endogenous (atopic) eczema arises from a hereditary or constitutional tendency to develop hypersensitivity reactions. Eczema responds to topical therapy. Since a characteristic of eczema is dry skin, the use of emollients is particularly important. Intensive use will reduce the need for topical corticosteroids.

Topical steroids

➢ Steroids have been used in dermatology to relieve itching and suppress inflammation since 1952 and remain in common use for a variety of skin problems, including psoriasis, eczema and other types of dermatitis.

Psoriasis

➢ Psoriasis is one of the common skin disorders. Occurring equally in men and women of any age, its onset is usually in early adult life. Treatment comprises the use of ointments and pastes, oral systemic drugs or various forms of UV light therapy. Calcipotriol is a man-made form of vitamin D and is the first-line treatment of mild to moderate plaque psoriasis. Pimecrolimus and tacrolimus are new drugs used to treat psoriasis. Both are topical immunomodulators. When applied to the skin, they exert a powerful anti-inflammatory effect.

Acne

➢ Treatment of acne includes anti-comedonal agents, topical antimicrobials, retinoids and occasionally anti-androgen preparations. Steroids should not be used.

➢ A newer concept is the blocking of the activity of the androgen-metabolizing enzymes in the skin or in the sebaceous glands themselves. Such agents are called anti-androgens.

Calculations

1 How much malathion is in a 0.5% solution?

2 If you use a cream containing betamethasone 0.1 per cent weight by weight, how many mg of betamethasone will each g of the cream contain?

3 The patient is applying a cream that has a 2.5 per cent active ingredient. How much active ingredient is in a tube which contains 5g?

4 How would you express 1 in 50 as a percentage?

5 What is 0.5 per cent as a proportion?

6 A patient is to use a solution of 0.05 per cent. What is the strength of this solution in mg/ml?

7 A patient has been prescribed erythromycin 500mg four times a day for severe acne. You only have 250mg tablets. How many of these tablets are required to complete a seven-day course?

8 An adult female patient has eczema for which some cream has been prescribed. She needs to apply 15g to both hands. How many finger tip units will this patient apply in 24 hours?

9 A patient has a rash all over her body and needs some ointment prescribing. She requires: face 30g; both hands 50g; scalp 100g; both arms 200g; both legs 200g; trunk 400g; groin 25g. How much (in kg) does she need in total?

10 A 1 per cent solution is required but the only available strength is 10 per cent. How much of this will be required to produce 50ml of 1 per cent solution and how much diluent?

For further assistance with calculations, please see Meriel Hutton's book *Essential Calculation Skills for Nurses, Midwives and Healthcare Practitioners* (Open University Press 2009).

Multiple choice questions

1 Which of the following is the mainstay of eczema treatment?

a) Eteroids
b) Antibiotics
c) Zinc bandages
d) Emollients

2 Dithranol is used in which skin condition?

a) Eczema
b) Warts
c) Psoriasis
d) Acne

3 In which of the following conditions would you expect to use a steroid cream?

a) Eczema
b) General skin health
c) Acne
d) Warts

4 Topical retinoids are

a) Derived from vitamin A
b) Derived from vitamin D
c) Derived from coal tar
d) Derived from shale

5 The normal pH of skin is

a) 5.5
b) 4.8
c) 7.5
d) 6.4

6 Emollients are preparations which when used generously and frequently

a) Draw water towards them
b) Prevent water loss from the skin
c) Clog or block the pores
d) Absorb UV light

7 Drugs first have to penetrate which layer to be absorbed?

a) Granular layer
b) Stratum corneum layer
c) Prickle layer
d) Basal layer

8 The normal process of maturation and shredding is called orthokeratosis which takes several weeks. In which skin disorder is this reduced to 8–10 days?

a) Psoriasis
b) Acne
c) Eczema
d) Scabies

←

9 In which skin condition would you come across open and closed comedomes?

a) Eczema
b) Psoriasis
c) Warts
d) Acne

10 One of the newer, non-steroidal treatments for eczema is

a) Betnovate ointment
b) Hydrocortisone cream
c) Tacrolimus ointment
d) Minoxidil

Recommended further reading

Barber, P. and Robertson, D. (2012) *Essentials of Pharmacology for Nurses*, 2nd edn. Maidenhead: Open University Press.

Beckwith, S. and Franklin, P. (2007) *Oxford Handbook of Nurse Prescribing*. Oxford: Oxford University Press.

Brenner, G.M. and Stevens, C.W. (2009) *Pharmacology*, 3rd edn. Philadelphia, PA: Saunders Elsevier.

Charman, C. and Lawton, S., (2006) *Eczema: What Really Works?* London: Robinson Publishing.

Clayton, B.D. (2009) *Basic Pharmacology for Nurses*, 15th edn. St Louis, MO: Mosby Elsevier.

Coben, D. and Atere-Roberts, E. (2005) *Calculations for Nursing and Healthcare*, 2nd edn. Basingstoke: Palgrave Macmillan.

Downie, G., Mackenzie, J. and Williams, A. (2007) *Pharmacology and Medicines Management for Nurses*, 4th edn. Edinburgh: Churchill Livingstone.

Gatford, J.D. and Phillips, N. (2006) *Nursing Calculations*, 7th edn. Edinburgh: Churchill Livingstone Elsevier.

Greenstein, B. (2009) *Clinical Pharmacology for Nurses*, 18th edn. Edinburgh: Churchill Livingstone.

Hutton, M. (2009) *Essential Calculation Skills for Nurses, Midwives and Healthcare Practitioners*. Maidenhead: Open University Press.

Karch, A.M. (2008) *Focus on Nursing Pharmacology*, 4th edn. Philadelphia, PA: Lippincott Williams & Wilkins.

Lapham, R. and Agar, H. (2009) *Drug Calculations for Nurses: A Step-by-step Approach*, 3rd edn. London: Arnold.

Lawton, S. (2007) Skin barrier function and the use of emollient in dermatological nursing, *British Journal of Nursing*, 16(12): 712–19.

NICE (National Institute for Health and Clinical Excellence) (2008) *Atopic Eczema in Children: Stepped Care Plan for Managing Atopic Eczema in Children*. London: NICE.

O'Brien, S.C., Lewis, J.B. and Cunliffe, W.J. (1998) *The Leeds Revised Acne Grading System*. Leeds: University of Leeds.

Page, C., Curtis, M., Walker, M. and Hoffman, B. (2006) *Integrated Pharmacology*, 3rd edn. Edinburgh: Mosby Elsevier.

Ritchie, J. (2008) *Muscles, Bones and Skin*, 3rd edn. Edinburgh: Mosby Elsevier.

Simonson, T., Aarbakke, J., Kay, I., Coleman, I., Sinnott, P. and Lyssa, R. (2006) *Illustrated Pharmacology for Nurses*. London: Hodder Arnold.

Starkings, S. and Krause, L. (2010) *Passing Calculation Tests for Nursing Students*. Exeter: Learning Matters.

Drugs used to treat withdrawal

9

Chapter contents

Learning objectives

After studying this chapter you should be able to:

- Describe the role of reward pathways in the misuse of drugs/substances.
- Outline the extent of alcohol misuse in the UK.
- Explain the mode of action of medicines used in treating alcohol misuse.
- Describe the effects of smoking on the body.
- Demonstrate an understanding of the medicines used in helping smoking cessation.
- List the symptoms of opioid withdrawal.
- Discuss the types of drugs that are used in the treatment of opioid withdrawal.
- Correctly solve a number of drug calculations with regard to medicines used in the treatment of withdrawal from alcohol, nicotine and opioids.

Introduction

Drug addiction is a major problem in the UK and is caused by a variety of factors. Heroin, cocaine, cannabis and ecstasy are just a few of the many substances which are misused on a regular basis. They have a high profile and are seen as contributors to many of the problems in society today.

However, there are other, less obvious forms of drug addiction – for example, legal drugs such as alcohol, cigarettes and caffeine. These are used by many people on a recreational basis and in the case of alcohol and caffeine are seen as socially acceptable. Yet they can have far-reaching effects. Misuse can cause serious, long-term damage both mentally and physically, not to mention the social and emotional consequences. Drug misuse is one of the major forms of addiction in the UK and causes untold misery to many people. It doesn't just affect the addict: it also encompasses their families, friends, colleagues and the authorities.

Addiction is a chronic, often relapsing brain disease that causes compulsive drug-seeking and use, despite harmful consequences to the individual and those around them. It is a brain disease because the abuse of drugs leads to changes in the structure and function of the brain. Although it is true that for most people the initial decision to take drugs is voluntary, over time the changes in the brain caused by repeated drug abuse can affect a person's self-control and ability to make sound decisions, and at the same time send intense impulses to take drugs.

It is because of these changes in the brain that it is so challenging for a person who is addicted to stop abusing drugs. Fortunately, there are treatments that help people to counteract addiction's powerful disruptive effects and regain control. Combining addiction treatment medications, if available, with behavioural therapy is the best way to ensure success for most patients. Treatment approaches that are tailored to each patient's drug abuse patterns and any co-occurring medical, psychiatric and social problems can lead to sustained recovery and a life without drug abuse.

Similar to other chronic, relapsing diseases, such as diabetes, asthma or heart disease, drug addiction can be managed successfully. And, as with other chronic diseases, it is not uncommon for a person to relapse and begin abusing drugs again. Relapse, however, does not signal failure – rather, it indicates that treatment should be reinstated, adjusted, or that alternative treatment is needed to help the individual regain control and recover.

Reward pathways

Drugs are chemicals that tap into the brain's communication system and disrupt the way nerve cells normally send, receive and process information. There are at least two ways that drugs are able to do this: (1) by imitating the brain's natural chemical messengers, and/or (2) by overstimulating the 'reward circuit' of the brain.

Some drugs, such as marijuana and heroin, have a similar structure to chemical messengers, called neurotransmitters, which are naturally produced by the brain. Because of this similarity, these drugs are able to 'fool' the brain's receptors and activate nerve cells to send abnormal messages.

Other drugs, such as cocaine or methamphetamine, can cause the nerve cells to release abnormally large amounts of natural neurotransmitters, or prevent the normal recycling of these brain chemicals, which is needed to shut off the signal between neurons. This disruption produces a greatly amplified message that ultimately disrupts normal communication patterns.

Nearly all drugs, directly or indirectly, target the brain's reward system by flooding the circuit with dopamine. Dopamine is a neurotransmitter present in regions of the brain that control movement, emotion, motivation and feelings of pleasure. The overstimulation of this system, which normally responds to natural behaviours that are linked to survival (eating, spending time with loved ones, etc.), produces euphoric effects in response to the drugs. This reaction sets in motion a pattern that 'teaches' people to repeat the behaviour of abusing drugs.

As a person continues to abuse drugs, the brain adapts to the overwhelming surges in dopamine by producing less dopamine or by reducing the number of dopamine receptors in the reward circuit. As a result, dopamine's impact on the reward circuit is lessened, reducing the abuser's ability to enjoy the drugs. This decrease compels those addicted to drugs to keep abusing drugs in order to attempt to bring their dopamine function back to normal. They may now require larger amounts of the drug than they first did to achieve the dopamine high – an effect known as tolerance.

Long-term abuse causes changes in other brain chemical systems and circuits as well. Glutamate is a neurotransmitter that influences the reward circuit and the ability to learn. When the optimal concentration of glutamate is altered by drug abuse, the brain attempts to compensate, which can impair cognitive function. Drugs of abuse facilitate unconscious (conditioned) learning, which leads the user to experience uncontrollable cravings when they see a place or person they associate with the drug experience, even when the drug itself is not available. Brain imaging studies of drug-addicted individuals show changes in areas of the brain that are critical to judgement, decision-making, learning and memory, and behaviour control. Together, these changes can drive an abuser to seek out and take drugs compulsively despite adverse consequences – in other words, to become addicted to drugs.

Alcohol misuse

Alcohol misuse is widespread in England and 33 per cent of men and 16 per cent of women drink alcohol at levels that are hazardous to their health. In 2007 there were 863,000 admissions to hospital in England due to alcohol misuse, and 6,541 deaths directly related to it. The majority of these deaths were due to alcoholic liver disease (NHS 2011).

The problem of alcohol misuse has been recognized by the Department of Health (DH) which embarked on a campaign to educate the general public about the implications of drinking too much. The first step was to introduce the unit measurement of alcohol and guidelines about how many units men and women can safely drink. Nearly one

in four adults in the UK risks their health by drinking more than the recommended daily amount of alcohol. On average, men drink nearly twice as much alcohol per week as women. One unit is equal to 8g, or about 10ml, of pure alcohol. The number of units of alcohol in any particular drink depends on its strength and volume.

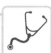

Clinical tip

The current recommendations for consumption are, that men should drink no more than three or four units per day. For women the number is lower and stands at no more than two or three units per day.

The recommended limits are lower for women than for men because women have different amounts of fat, muscle and water in their bodies. This affects the way women's bodies can cope with alcohol. Some experts think that women may develop liver disease at lower levels of drinking than men.

As a result of promoting a units-based scale, all alcoholic drinks sold in the UK must state on the label how much alcohol they contain. This is usually expressed as 'percentage alcohol by volume' (% ABV). The packaging of most drinks will also state the number of units of alcohol.

Despite the government's intervention there is a growing number of men and women who are dependent on alcohol in order to function. Equally, however, there are several drugs that may be used to help an individual combat their addiction to alcohol.

Disulfiram

For many patients, disulfiram (trade name Antabuse) is helpful in maintaining abstinence. This drug leads to an accumulation of the intermediary alcoholic metabolic product acetaldehyde when alcohol is consumed. Acetaldehyde is highly toxic and causes flushing, dyspnoea, palpitations, nausea and hypotension in the person who drinks alcohol while taking the drug.

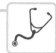

> **Clinical tip**
>
> Obviously a patient should be informed of the reaction they will experience before disulfiram is commenced. Some patients may only take 10 minutes to feel unwell. You must also be vigilant for any severe reaction to the medicine which may well require supportive treatment such as the giving of oxygen therapy. For this reason you will probably find that disulfiram is usually started in a hospital or a clinic setting and that it is supervised by a specialist in the field.

Disulfiram comes in 200mg tablets. The patient is often commenced on a dose of 800mg although you will find that this dose is lowered over a period of five days to a maintenance dose of 100–200mg daily. The patient should not normally take this medication for longer than a six-month period. You should also check that the patient has not ingested any alcohol for at least 24 hours before commencing this medicine.

Unusually, as part of its intended function this medicine produces extremely unpleasant side-effects even when only a small amount of alcohol has been consumed. Therefore it is very important to inform the patient that even mouthwashes that contain alcohol should be avoided when taking this medicine and they should also carry a card stating that they are currently taking disulfiram.

Given the reaction it produces, there are some circumstances (contraindications) under which it is not be advisable to prescribe this medicine. Examples are cardiovascular problems such as cardiac failure, coronary artery disease and hypertension, and any history of psychosis.

Discontinuation of disulfiram after its administration for several days or weeks still deters drinking for a three- to five-day period because the drug requires that long to be excreted. Therefore the patient should be advised not to drink alcohol for at least a week following discontinuation of the therapy.

Benzodiazepines

When heavy or frequent drinkers suddenly decide to quit they go through a process that is commonly called doing 'cold turkey'. They will experience some physical withdrawal symptoms, which can range from the mildly annoying to the severe and even life-threatening.

The severity of these withdrawal symptoms is usually dependent on how *chemically dependent* the patient has become. Those who drink heavily on a daily basis will have developed a high level of dependence, but even those who drink daily, but not heavily, and those who drink heavily but not daily, can become chemically dependent upon alcohol.

When someone who has become alcohol dependent decides to stop drinking, they will experience some level of physical discomfort. For this reason, it is extremely difficult for them to merely stop drinking on their own without assistance and support.

Alcohol withdrawal can be extremely unpleasant. Symptoms vary from person to person, but most people will experience some negative symptoms if they try to stop drinking after long-term use. Mild to moderate symptoms include headache, nausea, vomiting, insomnia, rapid heart rate, abnormal movements, anxiety, depression and fatigue. Severe symptoms include hallucinations, fever and convulsions (known as *delirium tremens* – DTs). Most people undergoing alcohol detoxification do not require hospitalization, but in severe cases it may be necessary.

Since their introduction in the 1960s, benzodiazepines have been the drug of choice for treating severe cases of alcohol withdrawal. They are discussed in Chapter 8 of *Essentials of Pharmacology for Nurses* in relation to mental health (Barber and Robertson 2012). They are a class of psychoactive drugs that work to slow down the central nervous system by activating gamma-aminobutyric acid (GABA) receptors. This provides a variety of useful tranquilizing effects. Aside from relieving symptoms of alcohol withdrawal, benzodiazepines are also commonly prescribed to treat insomnia, muscle spasms, involuntary movement disorders, anxiety disorders and convulsive disorders.

The most common regimen for treating alcohol withdrawal involves three days of long-acting benzodiazepines on a fixed schedule with additional medication available 'as needed'. The two most commonly prescribed benzodiazepines are chlordiazepoxide and diazepam. Chlordiazepoxide is preferred for its superior anticonvulsant capabilities, while diazepam is preferred for its safety against overdose with alcohol. Short-acting benzodiazepines like oxazepam and lorazepam are less frequently used for treating alcohol withdrawal.

Compared to other drugs, benzodiazepines are the safest and most effective method for treating difficult alcohol withdrawal. However, they do come with their own potential for dependence and abuse. Ironically, symptoms of benzodiazepine withdrawal are quite similar to those of alcohol withdrawal. Tapering off dosage is the best way to prevent serious withdrawal symptoms. For example, chlordiazepoxide 10–50mg may be given up to four times daily on initiating treatment but this will gradually reduce over a 7–14-day period. To avoid such complications, benzodiazepines are only recommended for short-term treatment of alcohol withdrawal.

Clomethiazole

Clomethiazole (chlormethiazole) is a sedative and hypnotic (sleep-inducing) agent that is widely used in treating and preventing the symptoms of acute alcohol withdrawal. The drug is structurally related to thiamine (vitamin B1) but acts like a sedative, hypnotic, muscle relaxant and anticonvulsant. You may have come across this drug in other situations since it can be used to treat agitation, restlessness, short-term insomnia and Parkinson's disease in the elderly. The brand name is Heminevrin.

The drug comes either in a capsule form or as a syrup. It works in a similar way to the benzodiazepines in that it enhances the action of the neurotransmitter GABA within the central nervous system. The GABA is the major inhibitory neurotransmitter in the brain and produces anxiolytic, anticonvulsant, sedative and hypnotic effects. Clomethiazole also inhibits the enzyme alcohol dehydrogenase, which is responsible for breaking down alcohol in the body. This slows the rate of elimination of alcohol which helps to relieve the sudden effects of alcohol withdrawal.

This medicine may cause drowsiness. Therefore the patient should be warned not to drive or operate machinery. Alcohol should be avoided as its effects are enhanced by this medicine. Tolerance and dependence readily occur. 'Tolerance' means that less effect is achieved from the same dose. 'Dependence' means that the patient finds it very difficult to stop using the medicine. As a result, abrupt withdrawal may result in serious problems. Finally, this medicine should not be used for more than nine days when treating alcohol withdrawal.

Clomethiazole is particularly toxic and dangerous in overdose, which can be potentially fatal.

Acamprosate

Acamprosate (brand name Campral) is a drug that has been shown to double abstinence rates in people receiving treatment for alcohol dependence. It is said to increase the likelihood of abstinence from 10 to 20 per cent and at best up to 40 per cent.

Although its mechanism of action is not clearly understood, acamprosate appears to block the excitatory activity in the brain of N-methyl D-aspartate (NMDA). This neurotransmitter is thought to be important in learning and memory. Acamprosate also enhances the inhibitory system (GABA). While it has been known as an 'anticraving' drug, the evidence is less conclusive about this as a major effect.

Acamprosate is considered when somebody is struggling to maintain abstinence and describes anxiety as a feature of their difficulties in remaining sober. Any underlying anxiety disorder will be appropriately treated, but in addition acamprosate will be considered. If somebody describes 'craving' and it is described as a desire to get a 'high' or 'buzz' from alcohol, acamprosate is less likely to be considered.

Acamprosate has been shown to be effective alongside psychosocial treatment and not in isolation. Patients should therefore not generally be offered the drug in the absence of receiving psychological support for their addiction (e.g. counselling, Alcoholics Anonymous). The drug has been shown to increase the number of 'dry days' in somebody trying to achieve abstinence. Importantly, however, it has been shown to reduce the number of drinks and number of days drinking in somebody who lapses. Patients have reported that they do not need as much alcohol to achieve the same level of satisfaction (this may be because alcohol and acamprosate appear to have similar effects on the brain).

Acamprosate appears to have a neuro-protective effect in that the number of brain cells that die during alcohol detoxification can be reduced by taking this drug. Interestingly, the same effect is not reproduced with diazepam, suggesting that benzodiazepines may prevent seizures but not brain damage. Therefore acamprosate may be started as part of an alcohol detoxification programme. However, you will not find that all alcohol clinics offer this drug routinely as part of a detoxification programme.

Currently there are no clear guidelines as to which patients may be more likely to benefit than others from receiving this medicine, although women and those that are more anxious may respond better. Acamprosate is less likely to be effective in those with cognitive damage.

The drug is given as two tablets (333mg each) three times a day for those that weigh 60kg or more. If less than 60kg, two tablets should be taken in the morning, one at midday and one at night. If fit and well, no specific blood tests need to be conducted.

Acamprosate is a very safe drug and side-effects are generally minimal and transient in nature. Gastrointestinal (GI) problems such as diarrhoea and nausea are the most common, but rarely prevent continuation with the drug. The contraindication to prescribing is currently only in those that have severe liver damage.

There are no absolute guidelines as to how long acamprosate should be prescribed, although the British National Formulary (BNF) recommends that it should not be taken for longer than a year. There is no clear evidence as to how much benefit is maintained after stopping the drug. However, it

would seem reasonable to suggest that if somebody is able to gain enough skills to remain abstinent while taking acamprosate, then they are more likely to remain abstinent.

Some areas of practice that you visit keep patients under monthly assessment and certainly would consider keeping them on acamprosate for one year before discussing its withdrawal if the patient was still abstinent. The difficulties arise when somebody is continually relapsing while taking acamprosate; in such cases generally the medicine would be stopped.

Cigarette smoking

Tobacco products have been used for thousands of years, and the key active psychopharmacological ingredient, nicotine, has been studied for almost 200 years. The annual cost of smoking to the National Health Service (NHS) in England soared from £1.7 billion a year in 1998 to £2.7 billion in 2008. However, the cost of smoking to the NHS would have risen even more – to more than £3 billion a year – if government action, health education and changing social attitudes had not led over the last decade to a fall in the total number of smokers from nearly 12 million to just over 9 million (Cancer Research UK 2011). From this perspective alone it is obvious that nurses should have an understanding of the treatments used in helping people give up the habit.

Nicotine is the tobacco plant's natural protection from being eaten by insects, and was widely used as an insecticide in the past. Nicotine is a toxin that, it has been suggested, is drop for drop more lethal than strychnine or diamondback rattlesnake venom, and three times deadlier than arsenic. However, in low concentrations (an average cigarette yields about 1mg of absorbed nicotine) the substance acts as a stimulant and is the main factor responsible for the dependence-forming properties of tobacco smoking.

Amazingly, by chance, this natural insecticide's shape is so similar to the neurotransmitter acetylcholine that once inside the brain it fits a host of chemical locks, permitting it direct and indirect control over the flow of more than 200 neurochemicals. When nicotine enters the body, it is distributed quickly through the bloodstream and can cross the blood-brain barrier (BBB). On average it takes about seven seconds for the substance to reach the brain when inhaled. So despite the coughing, dizziness and nausea associated with your first inhalation of a cigarette, within seconds it is affecting your acetylcholine receptors and stimulating your reward pathways by releasing dopamine. That is why people go back for more.

Apart from the effects of dopamine in the brain, the role of nicotine is fairly complex. By binding to nicotinic acetylcholine receptors, nicotine increases the levels of several neurotransmitters. It is thought that increased levels of dopamine in the reward pathways of the brain are responsible for the euphoria, relaxation and eventual addiction caused by nicotine consumption. Nicotine also brings about changes in enzymes that break down neurotransmitters at the synapses, therefore increasing their levels in other neuronal pathways.

Most smokers want to quit – in fact that is all some smokers talk about, but many fail to do so. Sadly, smoking is probably the single most avoidable cause of death and disability in the UK.

The health problems caused by smoking include cardiovascular and respiratory disease, cancer (e.g. lung, larynx, oesophagus, mouth, bladder, cervix, pancreas, kidneys), and infant deaths related to maternal smoking. Increasingly, the dangers of second-hand smoke, such as cardiac disease and lung cancer, are also being recognized by researchers and policy-makers.

In the long run, the most effective way to eliminate smoking-related illness is to prevent people from starting to use tobacco. For those who already smoke, discontinuing use is the best and surest option for reducing health risks. Drugs are available that increase the chance of a successful quit attempt.

Bupropion hydrochloride

In the UK the brand name for bupropion hydrochloride is Zyban, which is a *nicotine-free* quit-smoking aid. Instead of nicotine, it contains the chemical bupropion. It works by boosting the levels of several chemical messengers in the brain. With more of these chemicals at work, the patient experiences a reduction in nicotine withdrawal symptoms and a weakening of the urge to smoke. More than a third of the people who take Zyban while participating in a support programme are able to quit smoking for at least a month. Zyban can also prove helpful when people with conditions such as chronic bronchitis and emphysema decide it's time to quit.

> **Clinical tip**
>
> One of the drawbacks of using Zyban is that about 1 person in 1000 suffers a seizure if they take it. For this reason, people with epilepsy and certain other disorders should never take the drug. This demonstrates why people should be discouraged from sharing medicines with friends and relatives. Only a doctor can decide whether a given medicine is safe for a particular individual.

Treatment begins while the patient is still smoking. Zyban needs about a week to reach an effective level in the body, so to improve the chances of success the patient should not attempt to quit until the second week of treatment. The patient should set a firm date for quitting. If they are still smoking after that date, their odds of breaking the habit will be worse. The patient should keep taking Zyban for 7–12 weeks.

It is possible to use nicotine patches along with Zyban; however, combining the two treatments can raise blood pressure, so it's important to inform the patient to tell their doctor if they plan to use both. The patient should be told to stop smoking while using a patch, because too much nicotine can cause serious side-effects.

The medicine comes in tablet form and should be swallowed whole, not chewed or crushed. If the patient misses a dose they must not be encouraged to take an extra tablet to 'catch up'. Instead they should miss the dose and take their next tablet at the regularly scheduled time. Side-effects are relatively mild and may include a dry mouth and a feeling of sleeplessness. The patient should be informed that these side-effects should disappear over a period of a few weeks. If the patient is having problems sleeping the dose may be lessened by the prescriber. The usual starting dose is one 150mg tablet in the morning for the first three days. After that, the patient should take one 150mg tablet in the morning and another in the early evening. The doses should be kept at least eight hours apart, with the maximum recommended dose being 300mg daily. Zyban can be prescribed for 7 to 12 weeks; however, the doctor may recommend continuing treatment for up to six months.

This medicine can trigger seizures in a small percentage of people. Zyban's seizure-triggering potential is greater in those with an eating disorder such as bulimia or anorexia, and in those undergoing abrupt withdrawal from alcohol, sedatives and tranquillizers such as chlordiazepoxide (Librium) and diazepam (Valium). This drug should also be avoided in patients taking drugs classified as monoamine oxidase inhibitor (MAOI). Fourteen days must be allowed to pass between taking an MAOI and commencing Zyban therapy.

Nicotine replacement therapy

Nicotine replacement therapy (NRT) is a way of getting nicotine into the plasma without smoking. There are a variety of products available and these include nicotine gum, patches, inhalers, tablets, lozenges and sprays. All are available from pharmacies and other retail outlets. They are also available on prescription.

NRT works by stopping, or reducing, the symptoms of nicotine withdrawal. This helps the patient to stop smoking, but without having unpleasant withdrawal symptoms. NRT does not 'make' the individual stop smoking. They will still need to have the determination to succeed in breaking the smoking habit.

Apart from causing addiction, nicotine is not thought to cause disease. The health problems from cigarettes, such as lung and heart disease, are due to the tar and other chemicals in cigarettes. So, taking NRT instead of smoking is one step towards

a healthier life. The dose of nicotine in NRT is not as high as in cigarettes. Also, the nicotine from smoking is absorbed quickly, and has a quicker effect than in NRT. So, NRT is not a perfect replacement. Withdrawal symptoms are *reduced* with NRT, but may not go completely. The risk of becoming dependent on NRT is small. About 1 in 20 people who stop smoking with the help of NRT continue to use the therapy in the longer term.

Patients considering NRT will first need advice from their doctor, practice nurse, pharmacist or stop smoking clinic. In discussion they will need to decide on which type of NRT will suit them best. The next step is very important: setting a date to stop smoking and commence NRT.

Clinical tip

Some people prefer to stop smoking at the end of one day and start NRT when they wake the following day. They should be informed that they must not smoke at the same time as taking the nicotine replacement as they will be increasing rather than decreasing the amount of nicotine available to the brain. The patient should also be told that the nicotine replacement is not a 'now and then' option.

The prescriber must make a judgement about how much nicotine the patient requires. Products with higher doses should be offered to individuals who smoke more than 18–20 cigarettes a day. It is recommended that NRT is established for at least 8–12 weeks for the best chance of stopping smoking long-term. Obviously the dose of NRT is typically reduced in the later part of the course, and then stopped.

The patient is more likely to stop smoking if they receive counselling or support while taking NRT. As indicated earlier, a doctor, nurse, pharmacist or dedicated clinic can provide such support. You may yourself have given up smoking with this level of support, or been involved in smoking cessation clinics while on your placements. The manufacturers of NRT often offer support such as telephone

Box 9.1 Support agencies for smoking cessation

quitsmoking.about.com
www.nice.org.uk/PH010
www.quitmasters.co.uk
www.smokefree.nhs.uk
www.smoking-cessation.org

counselling, tapes, internet sites or personalized written programmes. These details come on the packets of the various NRT products. Box 9.1 provides some useful web addresses to pass on to people who want to give up smoking.

NRT increases the chances of quitting smoking, and a combination of NRT with support or counselling may give the best chance of success. There is not much difference in how well the various types of NRT (examined in detail below) work. Personal preference usually determines which one is chosen.

Nicotine gum

Two strengths are available, 2mg and 4mg. The higher strength should be used if the patient smokes 18 or more cigarettes a day.

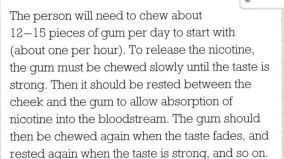

Clinical tip

The person will need to chew about 12−15 pieces of gum per day to start with (about one per hour). To release the nicotine, the gum must be chewed slowly until the taste is strong. Then it should be rested between the cheek and the gum to allow absorption of nicotine into the bloodstream. The gum should then be chewed again when the taste fades, and rested again when the taste is strong, and so on.

After two or three months the patient should be using the gum less and less. They may reduce the

chewing time, cut the gum into smaller pieces or alternate the nicotine gum with sugar-free gum. Gradually the gum should be stopped completely.

The disadvantage of gum is that some people do not like the taste, or they dislike always having something in their mouth. It may not be suitable for people who wear dentures.

Nicotine patches

A patch that is stuck onto the skin releases nicotine into the bloodstream. Some patches last 16 hours, which the patient wears only when they are awake. Other types of patch can last for 24 hours and are worn the whole time.

One problem with the 24-hour patch is that it may disturb sleep, but it is thought to help with the early morning craving for nicotine. Patches are also more discreet, and very easy to apply. The disadvantage is that a steady amount of nicotine is delivered, which does not mimic the alternate high and low levels of nicotine when a person smokes or chews nicotine gum. Skin irritation beneath the patch can also occur in some users.

The patches come in different strengths. The manufacturers normally recommend that the patient gradually reduces the strength of the patch over time before stopping completely. However, some research studies suggest that stopping abruptly is probably just as good, without the need to gradually reduce the dose.

Nicotine inhaler

A nicotine inhaler resembles a cigarette. Nicotine cartridges are inserted into it, and inhaled in an action similar to smoking. Each cartridge provides up to three 20-minute sessions. The patienr should use about 6−12 cartridges a day for eight weeks, and then gradually reduce over four further weeks. Inhalers are particularly suitable for those who miss the hand-to-mouth movements of smoking.

Nicotine tablets and lozenges

These are designed to be dissolved under the tongue (they are not swallowed). Nicotine is absorbed through the mouth and into the bloodstream. The main advantage with this route is that it is easy to use.

Nicotine nasal spray

The nicotine in the spray is rapidly absorbed into the bloodstream from the nose. This form of NRT most closely mimics the rapid increase in nicotine level that a person gets from smoking cigarettes. This may help to relieve sudden surges of craving. However, side-effects such as nose and throat irritation, coughing and watering eyes occur in about one in three users. As the nasal spray may cause sneezing and watering eyes for a short time after use, it should not be used when, or just prior to, driving.

Combination therapies

Combining different NRT therapies is an option, especially if the patient has particularly bad withdrawal symptoms. The common combination is to use an NRT patch (which gives a regular background level of nicotine) with gum or a nasal spray (taken now and then to top up the level of nicotine to ease sudden cravings). Evidence suggests that this kind of combination provides a small but significant increase in success rates compared with a single product. It is also thought that it is safe to combine NRT in this way.

As a rule, getting nicotine from NRT is much safer than from cigarettes because NRT does not contain the harmful chemicals in cigarettes. However, the following points may be relevant to some people.

In pregnancy NRT is likely to be safer than continued smoking and so its use can be justified in pregnant women who are finding it difficult to stop smoking. NRT products that are taken intermittently (such as gum, lozenges, sprays and inhalers) are preferred to patches to minimize the exposure of the unborn baby to nicotine. Liquorice-flavoured NRT products should be avoided because there is insufficient data on the safety of liquorice (glycyrrhizin) gums during pregnancy or breastfeeding.

If the patient is breastfeeding, the amount of nicotine that gets into breast milk is probably

similar whether the mother smokes or uses NRT. Breastfeeding within one hour of smoking or taking an NRT product can significantly increase the levels of nicotine in breast milk. Therefore, NRT products that are taken intermittently are probably best if NRT is used during breastfeeding.

If the patient is taking a drug called theophylline (used for some lung conditions) and stops smoking, the blood level of theophylline will increase because the chemicals in cigarette smoke interfere with this medicine. It is likely therefore that the dose should be be reduced, typically by about a third.

Varenicline

Varenicline (trade name Champix) is a nicotinic receptor partial agonist. A partial agonist activates a response but that response is less than nicotine would be. In this respect this medicine is different from the nicotinic agonist bupropion and NRT. As a partial agonist, it both reduces cravings for and decreases the pleasurable effects of cigarettes and other tobacco products, and through these mechanisms it can assist some patients to quit smoking.

Varenicline does increase the chance of quitting smoking (O'Dowd 2007). Studies have compared varenicline to a dummy (placebo) tablet in people who were keen to stop smoking. The results showed that, on average, about 21 in 100 people who took varenicline stopped smoking successfully. This compared to about 8 in 100 who took the dummy (placebo) tablets. In other words, taking varenicline more than doubled the rate of success.

Varenicline is generally thought to be a safe medicine for most people. However, it is a new medicine and so caution is advised. Varenicline was first licensed in the UK in December 2006 but it is not licensed to be used in people who are pregnant or breastfeeding, those under the age of 18 and those with severe kidney failure. It may also be used with more caution in people with mental health disorders.

Most doctors will only prescribe varenicline to people who really want to stop smoking as part of a 'stopping smoking' programme. Once prescribed the person should start taking the tablets a week before the 'quit date'. The aim is to build up the dose so that their body gets used to the medicine before the quit date. The usual advice is to start with 0.5mg daily for the first three days, then 0.5mg twice daily on days four to seven, then 1mg twice daily for 11 weeks. Each dose should be taken with a full glass of water, preferably after eating. So, ideally, after breakfast and after the evening meal.

The usual course of treatment is therefore 12 weeks. However, if the patient has failed to quit, an additional 12 weeks of treatment may be advised. Cessation of therapy should be discussed with their doctor. A short 'tapering off' of the dose over a week or so may be helpful because at the end of treatment, if the medicine is stopped abruptly, about 3 in 100 people suffer an increase in irritability, an urge to smoke, depression and/or sleep difficulty for a short time. These problems can be eased by a gradual reduction of dose.

Most people who take varenicline do not develop any side-effects, and, if they do, these effects are minor. The most commonly reported side-effect is nausea. This is often mild and tolerable. Other reported side-effects include insomnia, abnormal dreams, headaches and flatulence. These side-effects can be reduced if the tablets are taken after a meal with a full glass of water.

Because this is a relatively new drug it is important to inform the patient to report any concerns they may have while taking the medicine to their doctor. Suicidal thoughts and behaviour have been reported by patients taking varenicline. The patient should be advised to discontinue treatment and seek prompt medical advice if they develop depression or thoughts of suicide. Patients with a history of psychiatric illness should be closely monitored throughout their treatment with this drug.

Opioid dependence

Opioids are discussed in Chapter 3 of *Essentials of Pharmacology for Nurses* (Barber and Robertson 2012). Dependence on this class of drug is a medical diagnosis characterized by an individual's inability to stop using opioids even when objectively it is in their best interest to do so. The problem is so

large that as early as 1964 the World Health Organization (WHO) put together an expert committee on drug dependence and defined dependence itself as being a set of physiological, behavioural and cognitive phenomena of variable intensity, in which the use of a psychoactive drug (or drugs) takes a high priority.

Signs and symptoms of opioid withdrawal syndrome include yawning, sweating, lacrimation secretion (discharge of tears), rhinorrhoea (runny nose), anxiety, restlessness, insomnia, dilated pupils, piloerection (goose bumps), chills, tachycardia, hypertension, nausea/vomiting, cramp-like abdominal pains, diarrhoea, and muscle aches and pains. Unlike withdrawal from alcohol or benzodiazepines, opioid withdrawal is not life threatening. Emergence of withdrawal symptoms varies with the half-life of the particular opioid – within 6–12 hours after the last dose of morphine/hydromorphone/oxycodone or 72–96 hours following methadone. Therefore the duration and intensity of withdrawal symptoms can be variable and is related to clearance of the drug. Withdrawal from morphine is short (5–10 days) but more protracted with methadone.

Opioid dependence is a complex health condition that often requires long-term treatment and care. Treatment is important to reduce the health and social consequences of dependence and to improve the well-being and social functioning of those affected. The main objectives of treating and rehabilitating patients with opioid dependence are to reduce dependence on illicit drugs; to reduce the morbidity and mortality caused by, or associated with, the use of illicit opioids, such as infectious diseases; to improve physical and psychological health; to reduce criminal behaviour; to facilitate reintegration into the workforce and education system; and to improve social functioning. The ultimate achievement of a drug-free state is the ideal but is unfortunately not feasible for all individuals with opioid dependence, especially in the short term.

As no single treatment is effective for all individuals with opioid dependence, diverse treatment options are needed, including psychosocial approaches and pharmacological treatment. Relapse following detoxification is extremely common, and therefore detoxification rarely constitutes an adequate treatment of opioid dependence on its own. However, it is a first step for many forms of longer-term abstinence-based treatment. Detoxification with subsequent abstinence-oriented treatment and substitution maintenance treatment are essential components of an effective treatment system for people with opioid dependence.

The pharmacological options in treating a patient with opioid dependence will now be discussed.

Methadone

Opioids are painkillers (e.g. codeine, morphine and diamorphine – heroin) that work by mimicking the action of naturally occurring pain-reducing chemicals called endorphins. Endorphins are found in the brain and spinal cord and reduce pain by combining with opioid receptors. However, opioids also act in the brain to produce a 'high' (feeling of euphoria) and hallucinations. They can be both physically and psychologically addictive and people taking them long-term can become dependent on them.

Methadone is an opioid that is used mainly to wean people off their addiction to stronger opioids such as diamorphine and is prescribed as a substitute. By acting on the same opioid receptors as other opioids, methadone prevents the physical withdrawal symptoms that occur when these drugs are stopped. This prevents physical cravings for the drug. Over time, the dose of methadone is gradually reduced until it can be stopped completely.

Because methadone is an opioid it is in itself physically addictive, but it is less psychologically addictive than heroin because it does not produce the same 'high' or sense of euphoria. This is due to its effects on a different mixture of opioid receptors and the fact that it does not excite these receptors as much as diamorphine does. This makes it easier to gradually reduce the methadone dose until no physical dependence remains. However, while this all seems very simple and straightforward, in reality it is not, which is why so many people on methadone withdrawal programmes fail to 'kick

the habit'. Therefore, methadone substitution therapy must be used in combination with other medical, social and psychological treatments if it is to be successful.

Methadone substitution therapy is usually supervised by a GP and a team of people dedicated to dealing with alcohol and drug abuse. Some of you will have worked with such a team as a placement, or you may have come across one in other placement settings. Most GPs will refer the patient to a community drug team to be assessed. Following assessment, a member of the team will usually contact the GP quite quickly to recommend a dose of methadone, and a plan for follow-up. Some GPs who are specially trained may assess patients themselves and prescribe without the need for referral.

Clinical tip

Methadone is usually prescribed as a once-daily dose in liquid form. The patient will usually be asked to take it under the supervision of the pharmacist who dispenses the methadone to them. This means there can be no doubt about how much methadone the patient is receiving at each dose. This supervision may be relaxed after a few months of the patient taking a regular maintenance dose.

The aim of the substitution therapy is to prevent withdrawal symptoms. However, methadone can cause serious harm, or death, in overdose. Therefore, at first the doctor will prescribe a low dose to 'play safe'. An initial dose of methadone usually commences between 10–40mg although this can be increased if successful by 10mg daily. It is not recommended that an increase of more than 30mg is made within one week.

Methadone takes between two and four hours to reach peak effect and accumulate in the body. Thus the patient will not feel an effect for a few days. It may even take a few weeks to get to the correct dose which prevents all withdrawal symptoms. The patient should be asked to accept that they may have some, or partial, withdrawal symptoms until the correct dose is found. The 'correct dose' varies from person to person depending on how much heroin they are using and how their body deals with (metabolizes) the methadone. The patient should be asked to refrain from taking any street drugs or much alcohol when they are on methadone. All this requires patience in the early stages of treatment until an appropriate dose can be established. This in itself can be problematic for some addicts because the craving is so overwhelming.

However, once established on a regular dose, most people stay on methadone for a long time or even long-term. This is called *maintenance* and helps them keep off street drugs. Some people gradually reduce the dose and come off it. This is called *detoxification* or 'detox'. However, it usually takes months, and sometimes years, before most patients are ready to consider detox. It is often safer to stay on methadone than to detox before the patient is ready.

Driving becomes an obvious problem for people who have become dependent on opiates as their reaction times will be affected. The Driver and Vehicle Licensing Agency (DVLA) must be notified if the patient is dependent on opioids and their licence will be withdrawn. However, if the patient is on a supervised methadone programme, they may be allowed to drive again subject to annual medical reviews.

Pregnancy is another situation that needs thought if the mother is receiving methadone. Pregnant women have been treated with methadone for more than 25 years and neither methadone nor other opiates have been shown to directly cause birth defects. However, the baby may experience some side-effects from methadone. The most common are smaller-than-normal head size, low birth weight and withdrawal symptoms. As babies born dependent on methadone grow, they will usually fall into the normal range for size and development.

Some women ask about tapering off methadone while they are pregnant. However, medical withdrawal in pregnancy is not indicated or recommended. Medically, pregnant women have been safely tapered off methadone, but only on an in-patient basis where the foetus can be monitored for any distress. A pregnant woman should never be encouraged to detoxify herself. This can be very dangerous to the individual and their baby and put their recovery in jeopardy. It is far better to receive a maintenance dose and stick to it during pregnancy and it is not uncommon for a dose to be *increased* during pregnancy. This is because by the third trimester the amount of blood in the woman's body almost doubles, requiring a greater dose to keep mother and baby free from withdrawal symptoms. Ironically, an increase in methadone (if required) during this period can help to improve growth and reduce the risk of premature delivery. The key to a successful pregnancy when taking methadone is to make sure the individual is *stable* on their dose.

Buprenorphine

Buprenorphine is an effective, safe medication for use in the treatment of opioid dependence and is a valuable addition to the formulary of medications for treating this condition. It was licensed for use in opioid dependence in the UK in 1999. Buprenorphine has a low intrinsic agonist activity – it only partially excites the same opioid receptors as diamorphine. This means that doses of this drug produce a milder, less euphoric and less sedating effect than high doses of other opioids such as diamorphine or methadone. However, its effects are sufficient to prevent or alleviate opioid withdrawal, including a patient's craving for the drug.

Buprenorphine locks tightly onto certain opioid receptors called *Mu receptors* more tightly than diamorphine or methadone. Therefore, if prescribed in doses greater than 8mg it prevents these receptors from being used by other opioids such as diamorphine or methadone. As a result buprenorphine produces reduced opioid responses while at the same time reducing the effects of additional diamorphine.

Buprenorphine sublingual tablets are licensed for treating opioid dependence in the UK. They contain buprenorphine hydrochloride and are available in 400mcg (0.4mg), 2mg and 8mg strengths. The tablets are administered sublingually because this drug has poor oral bioavailability (i.e. it is inactivated by gastric acid and a high first pass metabolism). Initially the dose would be between 0.8–4mg as a single daily administration. This may then be adjusted according to the patient's response to a maximum daily dose of 32mg. However the usual maintenance dose is between 8–32mg. As with methadone the dose is normally supervised by a pharmacist.

Most of the unwanted effects of buprenorphine are similar to those associated with other opioids, and include constipation, headaches (common with this drug), sleeplessness, sickness and sweating. In addition many patients complain of a bitter taste. As with other opiates, side-effects vary from individual to individual, but are usually most prominent in the first few days of treatment.

Clinical tip

Subjectively, many patients on buprenorphine often report a 'clear head' response quite different from the 'clouding' associated with heroin or methadone use. Some patients find this 'clarity' uncomfortable whereas others may value it. This subjective experience may be a factor that influences patient choice.

As with methadone an assessment is essential to determine suitability for treatment. This should include urine drug testing to ascertain the presence of opioids. Patients entering treatment should have liver function tests and screening for blood-borne viruses (HIV and hepatitis A, B and C), although initiation of treatment should not be unnecessarily delayed while waiting for the results. Buprenorphine use, like methadone, will depend on adequate dosing and the concurrent delivery of non-pharmacological interventions that directly and indirectly address the underlying disorder of opioid dependence. As with methadone, buprenorphine can be associated with sedation, respiratory depression and coma when used in conjunction with central nervous system depressants such as alcohol, benzodiazepines, barbiturates, neuroleptics and tricyclic antidepressants. Therefore these should be vigorously discouraged by the prescriber.

Pregnancy is not a contraindication to the use of this medicine, rather it is a special warning. Trials suggest that it may be useful in pregnancy but there is as yet insufficient safety data to recommend its use. It has a similar incidence, compared to methadone, of neonatal abstinence syndrome (symptoms of drug withdrawal in the baby), but this tends to be less severe and needs less and shorter treatment. A pregnant patient on buprenorphine should be referred to a specialist and told that she can continue with the current treatment while at the same time being made aware of the facts. It is recommended that when the patient has given informed consent, this consent is documented in the medical and nursing notes.

Buprenorphine is an effective intervention for use in the maintenance treatment of heroin dependence, but it is not more effective than methadone at adequate dosages. Also, buprenorphine is not significantly different from methadone in its impact on other substance use (e.g. cocaine, benzodiazepines, alcohol). With similar outcomes, the choice between methadone and buprenorphine should be informed by other factors. There is limited evidence of the superiority of either medication and the decision as to which to use should be made in consultation with each patient after consideration of the relative merits.

Naltrexone

Naltrexone is an opioid receptor antagonist used primarily in the management of alcohol and opioid dependence. That means that the medicine locks onto opioid receptors, preventing opioids from stimulating them. You should not confuse it with naloxone (which is used in emergency cases of overdose rather than for longer-term dependence control). Both naltrexone and naloxone are full antagonists and will treat an opioid overdose, but naltrexone is longer-acting than naloxone making naloxone a better emergency antidote.

Naltrexone is sometimes used for carrying out what is called *rapid detoxification* regimens for opioid dependence. The principle of rapid detoxification is to induce opioid-receptor blockage while the patient is in a state of impaired consciousness, so as to weaken the withdrawal symptoms. Rapid detoxification can be carried out under general anaesthesia but this involves making the patient unconscious and requires putting a tube into their trachea (intubation) and external ventilation. A more popular choice is rapid detoxification under sedation. The procedure is followed by oral naltrexone daily for up to 12 months for opioid dependence management.

There are a number of practitioners who will use a naltrexone implant placed in the lower abdomen, and more rarely in the posterior to replace the oral naltrexone. This implant procedure has not been shown scientifically to be successful in 'curing' subjects of their addiction, though it does provide a better solution than oral naltrexone for medication compliance reasons. There is currently scientific disagreement as to whether this procedure should be performed under local or general anaesthesia, due to the rapid, and sometimes severe, withdrawal that occurs from the naltrexone displacing the opiates from the receptor sites. Therefore you are much more likely to come across the medicine being given over a much longer period of time.

Rapid detoxification has been criticized by some for its questionable efficacy in long-term opioid dependence management. It has also often been misrepresented as a one-off 'cure' for opioid dependence, when it is only intended as the initial step in an overall drug rehabilitation regimen. Rapid detoxification is effective for short-term opioid detoxification, but is approximately 10 times more expensive than conventional detoxification procedures. The use of naltrexone remains a treatment only for a small part of the opioid-dependent population, usually those with an unusually stable social situation and motivation (e.g. dependent health care professionals).

Naltrexone helps patients overcome urges to abuse opiates by blocking the euphoric effects. Some patients do well with it, but the oral formulation has a drawback. It must be taken daily and the dose usually commences as 25mg, increased to 50mg daily. However, in a patient whose craving becomes overwhelming there is nothing to stop them obtaining opiate euphoria simply by skipping a dose before resuming abuse. A preferable alternative for those likely to skip doses is a naltrexone implant, which may be surgically inserted under the skin. The implant provides a sustained dose of naltrexone to the patient, thereby preventing the problems which may be associated with skipping doses. It must be replaced every several months. The implant appears to be a far more effective means of treating heroin addiction than the oral formulation.

Lofexidine hydrochloride

This drug has a totally different mode of action from any we have discussed so far in this section on opioid dependence. Lofexidine is an alpha-2 adrenergic receptor agonist. Historically it was used in the treatment of high blood pressure as a short-acting anti-hypertensive. Today, however, you are more likely to come across it being used to alleviate physical symptoms of opiate withdrawal.

This drug has been used in opiate withdrawal since 1992 in the UK and is also commonly used in conjunction with the opioid receptor antagonist naltrexone in rapid detoxification cases. When these two drugs are paired, naltrexone is administered to induce an opioid-receptor blockade which attenuates the withdrawal symptoms and accelerates the detoxification process, while lofexidine is given to relieve physical withdrawal symptoms, including chills, sweating, stomach cramps, muscle pain and runny nose. As opiate withdrawal relief, lofexidine works to restore natural levels of noradrenaline and endorphins to pre-opiate addiction levels.

Some opioid detoxification programmes use methadone in decreasing amounts in their detoxification protocol while others use lofexidine. The drugs are chemically unrelated as are their physiological effects, although both are used as part of detoxification protocols. Whereas lofexidine cannot stop opioid withdrawal and merely eases some symptoms, methadone – being an opioid itself – will completely improve all withdrawal symptoms in a sufficient dose. Indeed, one suggested use for lofexidine is to ease withdrawal symptoms of *methadone* dependence.

While abstaining from opiates and taking lofexidine, effective detoxification can succeed in as little as 3 days, although the standard duration is 7–10 days. The initial dose of lofexidine is 800mcg daily, given in divided doses. This initial dose is increased in 400–800mcg steps until a ceiling is reached of 2.4mg daily in divided doses.

Case studies

① You are on a community placement working with the practice nurse. She is running a smoking cessation programme and asks you what alternatives are available as NRT.

● What would you say?

② Your placement is with the alcohol detoxification team. Your mentor wishes to know how much you know about disulfiram and how it is used in this field.

● What do you tell him?

Key learning points

Introduction

➤ Addiction is a chronic, often relapsing brain disease that causes compulsive drug-seeking.

Reward pathways

➤ Nearly all drugs, directly or indirectly, target the brain's reward system by flooding the circuit with dopamine.

Alcohol misuse

➤ Alcohol misuse is widespread in England.

Disulfiram

➤ This drug leads to an accumulation of the intermediary alcoholic metabolic product acetaldehyde when alcohol is consumed.
➤ Acetaldehyde is highly toxic and causes flushing, dyspnoea, palpitations, nausea and hypotension in the person who drinks alcohol while taking disulfiram.

Benzodiazepines

➢ Since their introduction in the 1960s, benzodiazepines have been the drug of choice for treating severe cases of alcohol withdrawal.
➢ They slow down the central nervous system by activating GABA receptors.

Clomethiazole

➢ Works to enhance the action of the neurotransmitter GABA within the central nervous system.

Acamprosate

➢ Shown to double abstinence rates in people receiving treatment for alcohol dependence.

Cigarette smoking

➢ The annual cost of smoking to the NHS has soared from £1.7 billion a year in 1998 to £2.7 billion in 2008.

Bupropion hydrochloride

➢ The brand name for bupropion hydrochloride is Zyban.

Nicotine replacement therapy

➢ There are a variety of products available to the individual such as nicotine gum 2mg and 4mg, patches, inhalers, tablets and lozenges, and nasal sprays, depending on patient preference.
➢ NRT products can be used in combination.

Varenicline

➢ A nicotinic receptor partial agonist.

Opioid dependence

➢ Emergence of withdrawal symptoms varies with the half-life of the particular opioid.
➢ No single treatment is effective for all individuals with opioid dependence.

Methadone

➢ Methadone is an opioid that is used mainly to wean people off their addiction.
➢ By acting on the same opioid receptors as other opioids, methadone prevents the physical withdrawal symptoms.

Buprenorphine

➢ Buprenorphine has a low intrinsic agonist activity.
➢ It locks tightly onto certain opioid receptors called Mu receptors.

→

←

Naltrexone

➢ Locks onto opioid receptors, preventing opioids from stimulating them.
➢ Should not be confused with naloxone.

Lofexidine hydrochloride

➢ Lofexidine is an alpha-2 adrenergic receptor agonist.
➢ It has been used in opiate withdrawal since 1992.
➢ It is commonly used in conjunction with the opioid receptor antagonist naltrexone in rapid detoxification cases.

Calculations

1 Disulfiram 800mg is to be given. You have 200mg tablets. How many will you give?

2 Acamprosate 666mg is prescribed three times per day. You have 333mg tablets. How many tablets would you give in a 24-hour period?

3 A doctor prescribes chlormethiazole 1g orally. You have a syrup containing 250mg in 5ml. How much do you give?

4 Chlormethiazole capsules contain 192mg. Convert this to mcg.

5 A person is taking Nicotinell chewing gum to help them give up smoking. They are taking the 4mg strength dose. The maximum dose is 60mg per day. How many pieces will be their maximum in a day?

6 Varenicline is prescribed as a 500mcg tablet. How would this dose be expressed in mg?

7 A patient is receiving buprenorphine 400mcg daily as part of their treatment for withdrawal from opioids. How many mg will the patient require over a seven-day period?

8 A patient has incrementally reached the maximum dose of lofexidine which is 2.4mg daily. The tablets come in a dose of 200mcg. How many tablets will they receive daily to meet this maximum dose?

9 A patient is initially prescribed methadone 0.04g daily. How many mg orally would you give?

10 An opioid-free patient has agreed to receive naltrexone on Mondays, Wednesdays and Fridays. They are prescribed 350mg per week. The tablets come as 50mg. Considering this, what dose per day would be the most logical to give?

For further assistance with calculations, please see Meriel Hutton's book *Essential Calculation Skills for Nurses, Midwives and Healthcare Practitioners* (Open University Press 2009).

Multiple choice questions

1 Nearly all drugs target the brain's reward system by flooding the circuit with

a) Dopamine
b) Serotonin
c) Acetylcholine
d) Noradrenaline

2 The current recommendations for alcohol consumption for men are

a) 0 to 1 units per day
b) 1 to 2 units per day
c) 3 to 4 units per day
d) 4 to 5 units per day

3 Disulfiram works by

a) Inducing sedation
b) Activating GABA receptors
c) Blocking dopamine receptors
d) Producing acetaldehyde when alcohol is consumed

4 Benzodiazepines help relieve alcohol withdrawal because of their actions on

a) GABA receptors
b) Dopamine receptors
c) Serotonin receptors
d) Acetylcholine receptors

5 Which drug blocks the excitatory activity in the brain of NMDA?

a) Disulfiram
b) Chlormethiazole
c) Acamprosate
d) Chlordiazepoxide

6 Which of the following drugs is used in nicotine withdrawal?

a) Acamprosate
b) Lofexidine hydrochloride
c) Methadone
d) Bupropion hydrochloride

→

7 Heminevrin is the trade name for which drug?

a) Bupropion hydrochloride
b) Chlormethiazole
c) Chlordiazepoxide
d) Acamprosate

8 Which drug is used in withdrawal from opioids?

a) Bupropion hydrochloride
b) Buprenorphine
c) Acamprosate
d) Chlormethiazole

9 Naltrexone is what we refer to as

a) An opioid receptor partial antagonist
b) An opioid receptor partial agonist
c) An opioid receptor agonist
d) An opioid receptor antagonist

10 Varenicline is a drug used in

a) Nicotine withdrawal
b) Alcohol withdrawal
c) Opioid withdrawal
d) All of the above

Recommended further reading

Barber, P. and Robertson, D. (2012) *Essentials of Pharmacology for Nurses*, 2nd edn. Maidenhead: Open University Press.

Beckwith, S. and Franklin, P. (2007) *Oxford Handbook of Nurse Prescribing*. Oxford: Oxford University Press.

Brenner, G.M. and Stevens, C.W. (2009) *Pharmacology*, 3rd edn. Philadelphia, PA: Saunders Elsevier.

Callow, T., Donaldson, S. and de Ruiter, M. (2008) Effectiveness of home detoxification: a clinical audit, *British Journal of Nursing*, 17(11), 692–5.

Cancer Research UK (2011) *Smoking Statistics*, www.cancerresearchuk.org/cancerstats/types/lung/smoking.

Clayton, B.D. (2009) *Basic Pharmacology for Nurses*, 15th edn. St Louis, MO: Mosby Elsevier.

Coben, D. and Atere-Roberts, E. (2005) *Calculations for Nursing and Healthcare*, 2nd edn. Basingstoke: Palgrave Macmillan.

Cox, S. and Alcorn, R. (1995) Lofexidine and opiate detoxification, *Journal of Mental Health*, 4(5): 469–73.

Downie, G., Mackenzie, J. and Williams, A. (2007) *Pharmacology and Medicines Management for Nurses*, 4th edn. Edinburgh: Churchill Livingstone.

Foster, J.H. (2004) The recognition and treatment of acute alcohol withdrawal, *Nursing Times*, 100(42): 40–3.

Gatford, J.D. and Phillips, N. (2006) *Nursing Calculations*, 7th edn. Edinburgh: Churchill Livingstone Elsevier.

Greenstein, B. (2009) *Clinical Pharmacology for Nurses*, 18th edn. Edinburgh: Churchill Livingstone.

Hutton, M. (2009) *Essential Calculation Skills for Nurses, Midwives and Healthcare Practitioners*. Maidenhead: Open University Press.

Karch, A.M. (2008) *Focus on Nursing Pharmacology*, 4th edn. Philadelphia, PA: Lippincott Williams & Wilkins.

Lapham, R. and Agar, H. (2009) *Drug Calculations for Nurses: A Step-by-step Approach*, 3rd edn. London: Arnold.

McClelland, G. (2005) How to manage opiate dependence and withdrawal, *Nursing Times*, 101(37): 30–2.

McLoughlin, C. (2005) Nicotine replacement, *Professional Nurse*, 20(7): 50–1.

NHS (National Health Service) (2011) Clinical knowledge summaries: alcohol misuse, www.cks.nhs.uk/patient_information_leaflet/view_as_a_leaflet. Patient information leaflet – Alcohol misuse.

O'Dowd, A. (2007) New non-nicotine drug to help smoking cessation efforts, *Nursing Times*, 103(24): 23–4.

Percival, J. (2005) Helping people to stop smoking: the role of treatment products, *Nursing Times*, 101(48): 52–4.

Simonson, T., Aarbakke, J., Kay, I., Coleman, I., Sinnott, P. and Lyssa, R. (2006) *Illustrated Pharmacology for Nurses*. London: Hodder Arnold.

Starkings, S. and Krause, L. (2010) *Passing Calculation Tests for Nursing Students*. Exeter: Learning Matters.

Complementary therapies and pharmacology

10

Learning objectives

After studying this chapter you should be able to:

- Show an awareness of the main branches of complementary and alternative medicines.
- Understand that the use of herbs and other plants is a constituent part of many of these.
- Show an awareness of the history of herbal medicine.
- Name some commonly used herbal remedies and their methods of use.
- Show an awareness of the conditions that may be treated by them.
- Understand that following simple guidelines when purchasing and using herbal remedies will make their use more safe.
- Understand how herbal medicines may be used both alongside standard western medical treatments and independent of them, but that concomitant use of some may cause side-effects, and that contraindications exist.

Introduction

You may be a little surprised at finding this chapter in a book dealing with pharmacology, but complementary and alternative medicines (CAMs) are increasingly used in Western health care, both alongside conventional medicines and independent of them. You may have made use of complementary therapies yourself. If so, you will be aware of the wide range available. If not, this chapter offers a brief introduction, and illustrates their use in relation to pharmacology.

The range, scope and use of complementary therapies

Modern Western medicine dates from the work of Hippocrates; however, Ayurveda and traditional Chinese medicine, both of which use herbal remedies in their treatments, are complete medical systems based on traditional principles thousands of years old. There has been an upsurge of interest in both of these in recent years and, ironically, they may now be considered truly 'complementary'.

The terms 'complementary' and 'alternative' are not easy to define. In the past, complementary therapies were regarded as an alternative to conventional Western medicine, and the two types were believed to be mutually exclusive. More recently, the term 'complementary' has been applied to those therapies which are used *alongside* conventional medicine. This can work well for many of the therapies outlined in this chapter. However, mixing herbal remedies (often self-prescribed) both with each other and with conventional drugs can pose problems.

It is beyond the scope of this chapter to do anything other than raise awareness of the many relevant CAM therapies available, so wider reading is recommended. A brief discussion of the history, development and use of CAMs in contemporary society is offered, focusing on those therapies which make use of herbs and other plants – particularly homoeopathy, aromatherapy and Bach Flower Remedies.

Understanding the true nature of CAMs takes time, patience and an open mind, as they are based on a philosophy of health very different from our own. Some are complete medical systems, while others form one or more branches of a wider system. Some make use of herbs and some do not. Complete medical systems include the ancient Ayurveda, traditional Chinese medicine, naturopathy, functional medicine, anthroposophic medicine, osteopathy and homoeopathy. What they each have in common is their ability to pay attention to the condition of the whole person (the holistic approach) rather than simply treating the disease. Often, this means looking at diet and lifestyle. There are literally hundreds of CAM therapies practised today which are, in the main, branches of the above. Several of these may be combined, and their use is expanding in areas such as palliative care (Parkes and Padmore 2011).

Popular therapies

Opinions differ as to what makes a CAM therapy 'popular'. We concentrate here on those most widely used. There are many others, and countless texts outlining what they involve. These should be consulted if more information is required.

Many therapies rely on what we might call a 'hands-on' approach – a tactile interaction between therapist and client. Massage and aromatherapy both make use of essential oils and are used to treat a variety of conditions. They are particularly useful in relieving the effects of stress. Often used alongside these, reflexology works on specific reflex points on the feet, hands or ears to relax, alleviate stress and relieve pain in the body,

> **Clinical tip**
>
> Even though a therapy may not involve the use of herbs directly, practitioners may advise on diet, suggesting herbal remedies to supplement the therapy.

Osteopathy and Chiropractic

Osteopathy and chiropractic are both manipulative therapies that concentrate on the musculoskeletal system. A chiropractor, however, focuses mainly on the spine and joints, while an osteopath will work with the structure and function of the whole body. Neither chiropractors nor osteopaths can prescribe medicines but many may give advice regarding the use of herbal remedies or appropriate over-the-counter medications.

Massage

Massage is a generic term for a variety of techniques which work therapeutically on the soft tissues of the body. There are various forms, including Swedish massage, sports massage and aromatherapy massage. Working on the skin, a masseur will manipulate muscle and connective tissue, aiming to enhance the function of these, promoting relaxation and well-being, easing tension and reducing pain. A carrier oil, often grapeseed or sweet almond, is used to facilitate free movement over the skin and limit friction. An aromatherapy massage will adapt these techniques to deliver essential oils, adding them to the carrier oil.

Aromatherapy

Aromatherapy is the systematic use of essential oils, extracted from a wide variety of plants and highly concentrated, to improve physical and mental well-being. Its use is very popular, both professionally and as a self-help therapy.

There are several ways of using these oils: massage, bathing, compresses or inhalation. They are believed to work through the absorption of minute quantities of the oil through the skin, and also through inhalation of the aroma. Essential oils should never be used orally or taken internally. Only tea tree and lavender are considered safe to apply to the skin neat and then only as directed. Examples of commonly used oils include lavender, tea tree, chamomile, eucalyptus, bergamot, sandalwood and rose. Many can be bought over the counter, but their safe use demands both knowledge and understanding. Oils can be used alone, or carefully blended in specific amounts. Some oils such as hyssop and clove are best administered by a qualified aromatherapist.

Essential oils can be adulterated. Buy wisely and store properly. Study the properties of each oil carefully. Some are known to react with certain Western medicines, some should not be used alongside homoepathic remedies. Others are contraindicated in certain conditions, particularly high blood pressure, epilepsy, pregnancy or breastfeeding. Some should not be used on children.

Homeopathy

Homeopathy works on the principle of 'like cures like': a substance which may cause symptoms leading to illness is used to alleviate those symptoms. For example, the homoeopathic remedy coffea is sourced from whole, unroasted coffee beans. Coffea is known to keep people awake and stimulated, so coffea is used to treat people who are mentally and physically overactive, and who may also have insomnia.

Remedies are prepared by diluting the active ingredient and shaking it in a specific way. The solutions produced are called *potencies*, expressed as 1c, 2c, 3c and so on. Some commonly used potencies are 6c, 12c and 30c, the high potencies being considered more powerful than the low ones. Many low potency remedies can be bought over the counter, and attention must be paid to using them correctly. When taking arnica, for example, the pills should not be touched nor taken after cleaning the teeth, smoking or after drinking tea, coffee or alcohol.

Homeopathic remedies are very popular and considered safe but their efficacy has been challenged. Homoeopaths must be statutorily registered, and are often doubly qualified, having other professional skills in medicine, nursing or pharmacy.

Bach Flower Remedies

Although others are available, perhaps the most widely used flower remedies are those developed by Dr Edward Bach in the 1930s. These make use of

38 flowers and plants, each designed to treat a specific human emotion. Aspen, for example, is used to treat anxiety. In addition to individual remedies, a blend is available under the name 'Rescue Remedy'. This is designed to deal with emergencies and crises when there is insufficient time to make a proper individual selection of remedies. Examples might be last-minute exam nerves or the aftermath of an accident. Such is the popularity of the Rescue Remedy that it is available in a variety of forms, including chewing gum. It may also be applied topically as a cream.

Clinical tip

Practitioners of many of these therapies have their own governing body. Some are regulated by statute, while others are unregulated.

Historical use of herbal medicines and other techniques

The use of herbs is as old as mankind. Herbal medicine as we know it may have its origins in the oldest complete medical system known to man, Ayurveda. This is thought to be at least 3000 years old, and is the traditional system of medicine practised in India. For the most part, Ayurveda works on a preventative basis, but, when people do become ill, a wide range of herbs and other treatments are used with the aim of helping the body heal itself. There has been an upsurge in interest in Ayurvedic remedies in recent years, and many books on self-medication exist. Traditional Chinese medicine, another ancient and complex system of healing, embraces the use of herbs, massage, nutrition and acupuncture alongside other hands-on techniques. Acupuncture is a therapeutic technique that involves the insertion of fine needles into specific points on the skin to keep the person in good health, as well as treating a wide range of disorders. Commonly used herbs include ginseng, ginger root and cinna-

mon. Many other ingredients may be incorporated, including insects, minerals and animal matter. Herbs are available as pills, and can be boiled to make teas, dried and ground into powder. Many Chinese medical clinics have opened in recent years, offering a range of treatments and herbal remedies.

Clinical tip

Chinese herbs have been known to contain impurities so should always be purchased from a reputable Chinese medical practitioner, and their source and quality guaranteed.

The modern context

There is also a long Western tradition of the therapeutic use of herbal preparations (often called 'medicines' but this can be a misleading term, given its Western connotations), their use being recorded by the ancient Greeks. As recently as 200 years ago, plants were the mainstay of 'traditional' medical treatments. It was the practice of herbalism and other therapies which made it possible for many of our conventional drugs to be created. Cocaine, morphine, anticoagulants and quinine are among the many drugs in use today based on plants and herbs. Aspirin comes from the bark of willow trees and digoxin from the foxglove plant. Many people, however, prefer to self-medicate with herbal remedies rather than take prescribed drugs.

Herbal medicine is a general term for the medicinal use of plant and other material. Scientists often try to separate a single active ingredient of a plant and produce it on a large scale in a laboratory. Herbal remedies, however, may contain dozens of different ingredients, as herbalists believe that all the elements are in balance within a plant and that keeping them together is important. Each different component is made more powerful through the 'synergistic' presence of the others.

Clinical tip

Grown and eaten as food or drink, herbs may bring beneficial side-effects of which we are unaware. Thyme is said to have mild antiseptic properties, to improve the immune system, promote perspiration and ease sore throats and coughs. Rosemary reputedly improves circulation, eases joint and headache pain and relieves cold symptoms. Mint relaxes the mind, can ease headaches, and, like ginger, can ease stomach and digestive problems, Peppermint aids the digestive system.

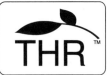

Figure 10.1 The THR symbol

Increasingly grown and harvested purely for medicinal purposes, the use of herbs may be said to have entered the medical mainstream. Such is their acceptance that a major high street chemist now offers a herbal alternative to each of its more orthodox pharmacological treatments. An interest in natural remedies has led to them featuring in mainstream television series.

Following European Union concerns about the growth in unregulated and dangerous products and the introduction of the European Directive on traditional herbal medicinal products (Directive 2004/24/EC), the UK established a traditional herbal registration scheme for traditional manufactured herbal medicines suitable for use without medical supervision. Operated by the Medicines and Healthcare products Regulatory Agency (MHRA), the scheme came fully into effect in 2011. Under this scheme any company manufacturing and marketing herbal remedies for sale in the UK must register its products with the MHRA. To receive registration, products must meet standards of safety, quality and patient information. Minor indications are based on evidence of traditional use rather than the normal requirement for regulated medicines to show efficacy. Following this assessment, products are given a THR (Traditional Herbal Registration) number comparable to the Product Licence Number (PLN) given to any licensed medicine.

A THR identifier for registered products, a small leaf symbol (see Figure 10.1), was also introduced, but its use was not made compulsory.

There are also plans to regulate herbal and traditional medicine practitioners under the Health Professions Council (HPC).

A person choosing to take a herbal remedy may self-medicate, follow the advice of a therapist or pharmacist, or consult a qualified nutritional/herbal practitioner. A medical herbalist is identified by the letters MNIMH (The National Institute of Medical Herbalists) or MCPP (The College of Practitioners of Phytotherapy). Phytotherapy is a medical treatment based exclusively on plant extracts or products.

If you choose to make use of a CAM, particularly if self-medicating, you should ensure you know the answers to the following questions:

- What is the origin of the product?
- What is its purpose? There are often several physical and psychological indications. Do any of these conflict with your proposed use?
- How should it be taken? With food, or should food be avoided? What is the correct dosage? What is the duration of treatment?
- If taking homoeopathic and Bach remedies, are the instructions clearly understood?
- What are the active constituents and is their potency guaranteed?
- Are there any adverse effects or contraindications?
- Are there any known interactions with other herbs, therapies or prescribed drugs?
- How should it be stored? What is the expiry date?
- Should it be stopped prior to surgery?

Clinical tip

The quality of a product can be affected by envirional factors such as climate and growing conditions before harvesting. Some have been known to be contaminated with pesticides, metals or other contaminants.

When might herbal remedies be of use?

Given that herbs can form the basis of complete medical systems it is difficult to give a comprehensive answer. However, in contemporary society they are often used to treat depression, hormonal problems, stress, or common, often chronic, health problems. Those having difficulty sleeping frequently prefer to use a herbal sedative, believing it to be a safer alternative to prescribed drugs. Herbs may be used to treat a variety of other conditions and are thought to be capable of the following:

- Relaxing tense tissues or organs such as the muscles or nervous system.
- Stimulating tissues or organs lacking tone.
- Acting as *astringents*, constricting over-relaxed tissues.
- Sedating overactivity in areas such as the bowel or nervous system.
- Promoting elimination of wastes and toxins from bowel, kidneys, liver, lungs and skin.
- Stimulating the body's defence mechanism and overcoming infection.
- Enhancing the circulation.
- Soothing mucous membranes while reducing irritation and inflammation.
- Regulating and promoting the secretion and action of hormones.
- Aiding appetite and digestion.

A herbalist will want to know the person's unique constitution, as well as the specific nature of the presenting complaint. When recognizing mild depression as a condition, a doctor would prescribe one of the many antidepressants commercially available. A herbal practitioner, while advocating the use of St John's Wort, may adopt a holistic approach, seeking out causes of the depression. As this remedy is readily bought over the counter, it is often self-prescribed.

Clinical tip

In spite of their many benefits, we must always be aware of the dangers of combining natural therapies such as herbs with synthesized western medicines. Some contraindications are discussed below. It is important to consult your health care provider before using any herbal supplement. Even if they do not know about a particular supplement, they can access the latest medical guidance on its uses, risks and interactions.

Choice of herbs, contraindications and drug interactions

The choice and range of herbal remedies is vast. Due to limited space, we discuss only a few of the most well known examples here. This information is intended to raise awareness of their use and provide a gateway for further reading. It is *not* to be followed as a therapeutic method.

In most cases, recommended dosage has not been given. This is intentional because dosage will vary according to the remedy and the condition being treated. Products will also vary in potency. Follow instructions for dosage carefully, and double check against other products you wish to use.

Clinical tip

The MHRA/CHM (Commission on Human Medicines) Yellow Card system allows you to report an adverse reaction to complementary remedies as well as other drugs and vaccines. Examples may be found in the British National Formulary (BNF) or online at www.yellowcard.gov.uk.

As their use grows ever more widespread, it should become standard practice for those prescribing medicines to enquire of patients if they are taking any herbal products. Choose your words carefully, as the patient may not think of CAMs as 'medicines'. A general rule is to advise patients who are taking any prescription drug to avoid herbal remedies. Similarly, a herbal practitioner should be advised if prescription drugs are being taken.

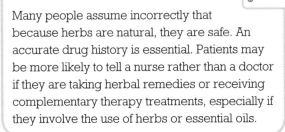

Clinical tip

Many people assume incorrectly that because herbs are natural, they are safe. An accurate drug history is essential. Patients may be more likely to tell a nurse rather than a doctor if they are taking herbal remedies or receiving complementary therapy treatments, especially if they involve the use of herbs or essential oils.

Echinacea

The purple flower and roots of this plant are used to treat a variety of conditions, aimed at improving the immune system and helping the body rid itself of infections. Unlike antibiotics, which directly attack bacteria, several constituents in echinacea, working together, are thought to stimulate the production and function of white blood cells, especially phagacytosis, making them more efficient at attacking bacteria, viruses and abnormal cells. Echinacea may also inhibit an enzyme (hyaluronidase) secreted by bacteria to help them gain access to healthy cells. It has been suggested that it increases the production and mimics the action of interferon, an important part of the body's response to viral infections such as colds and flu. Topically, it may be used to treat wounds.

Echinacea has an excellent safety record. However, it should not be used in progressive systemic and autoimmune disorders such as tuberculosis, connective tissue disorders and related diseases such as lupus. Echinacea is not recommended for use by people with multiple sclero-

sis, white blood cell disorders, or HIV/AIDS. Allergic reactions can occur and Echinacea may worsen metabolic control in some diabetic patients. Known side-effects include gastrointestinal (GI) disturbances, headaches and dizziness.

Garlic

Garlic is said to be one of the few herbs that has a universal usage and recognition. Crushing or chewing fresh garlic produces the sulfur compound allicin which, in turn, produces other sulfur compounds called allyl sulfides and ajoene (the latter having anti-clotting properties). Allicin is the principal biological active compound of garlic, and scientific evidence suggests that it is responsible for the many health benefits associated with this herb. It is a strong antimicrobial, and will combine with echinacea. Garlic may decrease blood cholesterol levels, prevent atherosclerosis and decrease blood pressure. It has been suggested it may have anti-cancer properties.

Garlic can irritate the digestive tract of very young children and some sources do not recommend garlic for breastfeeding mothers. Some individuals are allergic to garlic. It may exaggerate the activity of medications that inhibit the action of platelets in the body such as indomethacin and aspirin. There have been reports of a possible interaction between garlic and warfarin that could increase the risk of bleeding. When used with the sulfonylurea diabetic drugs, garlic may lower blood sugar considerably. Medications from this class include chlorpropamide, glimepiride and glyburide. If using garlic with these medications, blood sugars must be monitored closely.

Garlic may reduce blood levels of protease inhibitors, medications used to treat people with HIV, including indinavir, ritinavir and saquinavir. It is thought that garlic may behave similarly to statins (such as atorvastatin, pravastatin and lovastatin) and angiotensin-converting enzyme (ACE) inhibitors (including enalapril, captopril and lisinopril). It is not known whether it is safe to take this supplement in large quantities with these medications. This possible interaction has never been tested in scientific studies. Adverse effects may include nausea, hypertension or allergy. It may cause bleeding problems, and its use should be discontinued seven days prior to undergoing surgery.

Garlic is often taken as a supplement, either as a capsule or in a tincture. The recommended intake of fresh garlic is between 2g and 5g per day.

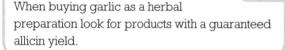

Clinical tip

When buying garlic as a herbal preparation look for products with a guaranteed allicin yield.

Ginger

You may think of ginger as flavouring a soft drink, or as the basis of a good curry, but it is much more than that – it is one of the most widely available and widely used herbal remedies. The root is used either fresh or dried and ground to a powder. The dried root of ginger contains approximately 1–4 per cent volatile oils. These are the active constituents of ginger and are responsible for its characteristic odour and taste. Anti-inflamatory and antiemetic, ginger is used in the treatment of fevers, respiratory problems, chills, colds and poor circulation, wind, colic and irritable bowel, nausea in pregnancy, motion sickness and following surgery.

A topical preparation of fresh ginger may be applied to relieve spasms, pain and cramps such as a stiff neck or shoulders. Ginger has been used in the treatment of parasitic infection because it contains a chemical called *zingibain* that dissolves parasites and their eggs. Made into a paste by mixing dry ginger powder with a little water or aloe gel and applied to the forehead it is said to aid sleep. Ginger can prolong the sleeping time induced by barbiturates. Use ginger with extreme caution if you are taking any kind of medication to induce sleep. The daily consumption of ginger root may interfere with the absorption of dietary iron and fat-soluble vitamins.

Ginger can increase the potency of anticoagulants (and aspirin), clopidogrel (Plavix), ticlopidine (Ticlid) or warfarin (Coumadin). Combining ginger with these medications could result in unexpected bleeding. Avoid taking ginger for two weeks prior to undergoing elective surgery or dental work. Avoid taking in acute inflammatory conditions.

There is some evidence that ginger may actually be helpful in alleviating gastritis and peptic ulceration, but care is needed in these conditions as any spice may exacerbate the problem. It should not be taken on an empty stomach as it can irritate the stomach lining.

Ginkgo Biloba

Also referred to as Ginkgo, it is best known for improving mental alertness, circulation to the extremeties and sexual function. Extracts of ginkgo leaves contain flavone glycosides and terpene lactones called *ginkgolides* and *bilobalides*, said to increase circulation to the brain and other parts of the body, as well as exerting a protective effect on nerve cells and vascular walls. Ginkgolides inhibit platelet-activating factor (PAF).

The benefits of ginkgo biloba extract (GBE) rely on the proper balance of these two groups of active components. These bioflavonoids are primarily responsible for GBE's antioxidant activity and ability to inhibit platelet aggregation. These two actions may help GBE prevent circulatory diseases such as atherosclerosis and support the brain and central nervous system. Stroke victims, those suffering from Alzheimer's disease or peripheral vascular disease may also benefit from taking ginkgo. It may also be used to treat premenstrual symptoms, tinnitus and altitude sickness.

Adverse effects may include GI upset or headaches. Those taking anticoagulants or anti-thrombotic medicines (including aspirin) should seek professional guidance before taking ginkgo. It should be avoided by those taking medication to prevent seizures or who have ever suffered a seizure. Ginkgo should not be taken two days before and one to two weeks after surgery or dental treatment to avoid bleeding complications.

Taking ginkgo is not recommended during pregnancy, breastfeeding or early childhood. Its use should be discontinued after three months if it is found ineffective. It combines well with ginseng.

> **Clinical tip**
>
> When buying ginkgo products look for the standardized guarantee for the active ingredients flavones glycosides (24 per cent) and terpene lactones (6 per cent).

Ginseng

Used for centuries in Asia and thought to enhance both mental and physical performance, there are three types of ginseng: Panax (also called Asian, Chinese or Korean), American and Siberian. All three are thought to stimulate the immune system. Ginseng is also said to lower both fatigue and blood sugar levels, particularly in those with Type 2 diabetes, to alleviate heart and lung disease and to reduce symptoms of stress and depression. Research has indicated that Panax ginseng may inhibit the growth of certain cancer cells.

Its active constituents are saponins – the ginsenosides. Ginseng may be taken as powdered dried root or as an extract. The level of ginsenosides can vary according to the preparation of these.

Adverse effects may include irritability, insomnia and GI disturbances. Ginseng should not be taken by those who are pregnant or breastfeeding, or who have diabetes or high blood pressure. It should be avoided by those taking anticoagulants, diabetic or heart medicine, diuretics, hormone replacement therapy (HRT) or painkillers. Tremor and mania have been reported when taken in conjunction with monoamine oxidase inhibitors (MAOIs).

Consuming large amounts of caffeine or other stimulants while taking ginseng can result in nervousness, sleeplessness, elevated blood pressure and other complications, as can taking higher than commonly recommended doses.

> **Clinical tip**
>
> Garlic, ginkgo, ginger and ginseng all promote bleeding and should not be used in conjunction with:
>
> - Anticoagulants (e.g. warfarin, heparin)
> - Anti-platelet drugs (e.g. clopidogrel, aspirin)
> - Non-steroidal anti-inflammatory drugs (NSAIDs – e.g. ibuprofen, naproxen).
>
> Neither should they be used in conjunction with other herbs that may promote bleeding. They should also be avoided by those about to undergo surgery or dental work.

Aloe Vera

Aloe Vera is one of the oldest and most widely used natural remedies. It has been said that its oil was used to embalm the body of Christ. A natural vegetarian source of vitamin B12, it has many documented uses but is best known for easing burns (when used topically), as an immune-system tonic and for soothing digestive tract irritations such as colitis, ulcers and irritable bowel syndrome (IBS). Its active compound, aloin, is obtained from the gel present in the leaf. Aloe Vera comes in a number of forms: natural gel, ointment, salve or lotion, liquid drink concentrate and encapsulated powder. Applied externally as a cream or ointment (which should contain a minimum of 20 per cent Aloe Vera), it restores skin tissues and may aid the healing of burns and sores. Taken internally, often to ease stomach disorders, the juice should contain at least 98 per cent Aloe Vera, but no aloin or aloe-emodin. For minor cuts and inflammation, the gel from the leaf may be applied directly to the wound.

Those using oral corticosteroids such as beclomethasone, methylprednisolone or prednisone should not over-use or misuse Aloe Vera. A potassium deficiency can develop and toxic effects may be experienced. It should be avoided by those who are pregnant, breastfeeding or menstruating.

A substance derived from the leaf (dried Aloe latex) and known as 'Bitter Yellow' is a laxative. This should not be confused with Aloe Vera, as they are very different, but it should also be avoided by those who are pregnant or breast-feeding.

Black Cohosh

This herb has some mildly sedative and anti-inflammatory effects and has been used to relieve nerve-related pain such as sciatica and neuralgia. It is thought to clear mucous and has been used to treat coughs.

The root may be eaten whole, ground into a powder or made into a tincture with water and swallowed. Black Cohosh contains several important ingredients, including triterpene glycosides such as acetin and cimicifugoside and the isoflavone formononetin. This is the active element in the herb that binds to oestrogen receptor sites, inducing oestrogen-like activity in the body. Extracts from the plant are standardized to contain 1mg of triterpine saponins per 20mg of the extract. It is used to treat painful periods, uterine spasms and the adverse symptoms of the menopause. Studies have found that the use of Black Cohosh can be as effective as HRT in the treatment of menopausal symptoms, thus offering a useful alternative for those women who cannot undergo HRT, or who have concerns about its long-term use.

There are currently no known interactions with other medications, although Black Cohosh may cause stomach upsets in some people. Due to its oestrogen-like effect, women who are pregnant or lactating should not use this herb, nor should people with hormone-dependent conditions such as endometriosis, uterine fibroids and cancers of the breast, ovaries, uterus or prostate. Women taking oestrogen therapy should consult a physician before using Black Cohosh. Its use has been thought to cause miscarriage, and there are concerns that long-term use may lead to liver-related problems.

Large doses may cause symptoms of poisoning, particularly nausea, vomiting or dizziness.

Cranberry

The juice from the berries is taken medicinally, although people often prefer to take cranberry in capsule or tablet form. This is thought to be more convenient, as several glasses of a high-quality cranberry juice would be needed to approximate the effect of the cranberry concentrate. If you choose to take it in liquid form it is important to ensure that the juice is pure, not one of the widely available blends.

Cranberry may be used to treat urinary tract infections, the most common cause of which is the bowel bacterium *E. coli*. Cranberry prevents this bacterium from adhering to the cells lining the wall of the bladder, rendering it harmless in the urinary tract. It is thought that a group of phytochemicals known as *proanthocyanidins* are responsible for this action.

Cranberries contain oxalates, chemicals which may contribute to the formation of kidney stones. Drinking large amounts of cranberry juice (more than about a litre per day) or taking concentrated cranberry supplements may increase the risk of developing this condition. Therefore, individuals who have or who have had kidney stones should not consume large amounts of cranberries, or use supplemental cranberry products.

The BNF advises that cranberry juice possibly enhances the anticoagulant effect of coumarins, and concomitant use should be avoided.

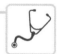

Clinical tip

Cranberry should not be used as a substitute for antibiotics during an acute urinary tract infection. Always seek appropriate medical advice.

Hawthorn

Hawthorn is a bush native to the British Isles and much of Europe. Its berries are used as remedies, either fresh, dried or as supplements. The leaves are occasionally used as an infusion. Hawthorn has been used to promote the health of the circulatory system and has been found to help strengthen the heart and stabilize it against arrhythmias.

Hawthorn contains active compounds with antioxidant properties. Antioxidants are substances that scavenge free radicals: damage compounds in the body that alter cell membranes, tamper with DNA and even cause cell death. Free radicals occur naturally in the body, but environmental toxins (including ultraviolet light, radiation, cigarette smoking and air pollution) can increase their number. They are believed to contribute to the ageing process as well as the development of a number of health problems, including heart disease. Antioxidants found in hawthorn can neutralize free radicals and help to maintain a healthy heart.

Hawthorn may be of benefit to those suffering from angina pectoris, atherosclerosis, congestive heart failure or hypertension. Hawthorn extracts standardized for total bioflavonoid content (usually 2.2 per cent) or oligomeric procyanidins (usually 18.75 per cent) are often used. Its bitter taste can be masked by mixing with sugar, honey, lemon or combining it in a herbal beverage blend.

Although non-toxic, hawthorn can produce dizziness if taken in large doses. Containing heart-affecting compounds that may affect blood pressure and heart rate, it should be avoided if colitis or ulcers are present. Those who are pregnant or breastfeeding should not use hawthorn, nor those using digoxin or phenylephrine.

Large amounts of hawthorn may cause sedation and/or a significant drop in blood pressure, possibly resulting in faintness.

Kava Kava

Once popular in the treatment of anxiety, insomnia, stress and feelings of restlessness. Its side-effects include hepatotoxicity and dermatological changes. Cases of hepatitis, cirrhosis and complete liver failure have been reported. Concerns led to its withdrawal in some parts of Europe and Canada, and, on 13 January 2003 Kava Kava was banned in England. This ban forbids the sale, possession for sale, offer, exposure or advertisement for sale, and the importation into England from outside the UK of any food consisting of, or containing, Kava Kava.

Milk Thistle

Historically, this herb has been used in Europe as a liver tonic and to treat a whole range of liver and gall bladder conditions. Its chemical components are now being shown to have a protective effect on liver cells. They are all flavones and flavo-lignins, the best studied being silymarin. This is made up of three parts: silibinin, silidianin and silicristin. Silibinin is the most active and is largely responsible for the benefits attributed to silymarin, which has been shown to reverse the effects of highly toxic alkaloids such as phalloidin and a-amanitin.

Widely used to treat alcoholic hepatitis, alcoholic fatty liver, cirrhosis, liver poisoning and viral hepatitis, milk thistle has also been shown to protect the liver against medications such as acetaminophen, a non-aspirin pain reliever. As the name implies, it promotes milk secretion and is perfectly safe as an aid to breastfeeding mothers. Women with hormone-dependent conditions such as endometriosis, uterine fibroids and cancers of the breast, ovaries or uterus should not take or use Milk Thistle plant extract due to its possible oestrogenic effects. Men who have prostate cancer should not take milk thistle without the approval of a doctor.

Silymarin stimulates liver and gall bladder activity and may have a mild laxative effect of short duration in some individuals. Applied topically, it has soothing properties. It may be used as a mouthwash to relieve blisters, or to soothe an ulcerated mouth.

Saw Palmetto

The berries of the saw palmetto are enriched with fatty acids and phytosterols. Extracts from these act to tone and strengthen the male reproductive system. A diuretic, urinary antiseptic and endocrine agent, Saw Palmetto berry tea used to be commonly recommended for benign enlargement of the prostate.

The constituents of Saw Palmetto are: essential oil 25 per cent, fixed oil consisting of 25 per cent fatty acids and 75 per cent neutral fats, sterols and polysaccharides (galactose, arabinose, uronic acid). The lipophilic (fat soluble) extract of Saw Palmetto provides sterols, and the fatty acids reduce the amount of dihydrotestosterone in the prostate.

Saw palmetto is thought effective in the treatment of benign prostatic hyperplasia (BPH). This is considered to be caused by testosterone accumulating in the prostate. The testosterone is then converted to dihydrotestosterone (DHT). The extract prevents testosterone from converting to dihydrotestosterone. It also inhibits DHT from binding to cellular receptor sites and so increases its breakdown and excretion. It is also believed to be useful in the treatment of colds and throat infections.

Those who are are pregnant or breastfeeding, have a hormone-sensitive cancer (breast or prostate), are using hormone-related drugs such as testosterone and oestrogen replacements, or are using warfarin should avoid taking saw palmetto.

Clinical tip

If you suspect that you are suffering from BPH it is important to see a doctor for a correct diagnosis. Do not attempt to self-treat with Saw Palmetto.

St John's Wort

St John's Wort is available in a variety of forms: dried herb capsules or extract, a water-based infusion, an alcoholic tincture and a cream or ointment. Its active ingredients (hypericin and hyperforin) influence neurotransmitters in the brain. It may boost levels of the so called 'feel-good' chemical serotonin, and is used for its antidepressant qualities.

Several bioactive agents are thought to contribute to this action, including proanthocyanidins, xanthones, phloroglucinol and flavonil derivatives. Hyperforin is thought, however, to be the most active. Having antibacterial and antiviral qualities, St John's Wort is used topically to treat wounds, burns, cold sores and haemorrhoids. Its oil is used as a treatment for sunburn. However, both oral and topical forms may make unprotected skin more sensitive to sunlight or artificial light in sun-tanning parlours. Some case reports have associated a higher risk of cataracts with possible eye sensitization to light when St John's Wort is taken. If using St John's Wort, sunscreen and eye protection should be worn when exposed to sunlight or artificial light used in sun-tanning.

Possible side-effects include GI upset, fatigue, dizziness, confusion and headache. Rare cases of serotonin syndrome (a potentially dangerous oversupply of serotonin in the body) have been attributed to taking St John's Wort. Uncontrolled serotonin syndrome may result in coma, seizures or death. Symptoms include confusion, euphoria, fever, hallucinations and an inability to control muscles.

St John's Wort should not be taken together with foods that contain tyramine, such as cheese, red wine, preserved meats and yeast extracts, nor should it be taken with the contraceptive pill, anti-epilepsy treatments or antidepressants. Anticoagulants and antifungals may also be affected, as may some antivirals. Its sedative properties may prolong the effect of anaesthetic agents, and its use should be stopped five days before any surgery.

Valerian

A widely accepted sedative, Valerian-based preparations are generally available in European pharmacies. The root has a variety of constituents, including essential oils, that appear to contribute to the sedating properties of the herb. Central nervous system sedation is regulated by receptors in the brain known as gamma-aminobutyric acid-A (GABA-A) receptors. Valerian may weakly bind to these receptors exerting a sedating effect.

Valerian is a much milder and possibly safer sedative than synthesized drugs (although cases of abuse have been known). Unlike Valium, it is not addictive, nor is it known to promote dependence. It can take two to three weeks of taking valerian extract before significant benefits in sleep are achieved. Due to this delayed onset of action it may not be an appropriate medicine for acute insomnia. On taking effect, however, it will promote natural sleep without any risk of dependence.

Valerian has been used in the treatment of blood pressure and as an anticonvulsant in the treatment of epilepsy. It will promote menstruation and is of benefit to the digestive system. It may help relieve colic and lower fevers, break up colds and heal stomach ulcers. Applied externally, it will relieve pimples and sores, but Valerian tea must simultaneously be taken internally.

Reported adverse effects include tremor, headaches, hepatic dysfunction and cardiac disturbance. Although no cases of drug interactions have been reported, animal studies have demonstrated that valerian can increase the effect of phenobarbital and benzodiazepines, and it should be avoided if taking these drugs. It should not be used by patients with liver problems. Valerian should not be taken in conjunction with sleep-inducing medication.

Dosage varies considerably, but a course of treatment should last no longer than three months. When stopping, the dose should be tapered, as acute stoppage may result in a benzodiazepine-like withdrawal.

Nutritional supplements and phytochemicals

Although not herbal remedies, these will often be found alongside them in pharmacies. Their use may also be recommended by a complementary therapist.

Evening Primrose Oil

The active ingredient of this essential oil is gamma-linolenic acid (GLA), an essential fatty acid. It is used to ease joint inflammaion and has been reported as easing aching joints in rheumatoid arthritis. Other conditions it may be used to relieve include mastalgia (breast pain) and atopic eczema. There are many more.

It may enhance any tendency to seizure and therefore, should be avoided by those suffering from epilepsy. As it may contain a small amount

of vitamin E, professional advice should be taken before use by those taking anticoagulants or medication to treat high cholesterol and blood pressure, oestrogen or other hormonal therapies. Women who are pregnant or breastfeeding should also avoid this oil.

Glucosamine and Chondroitin

These can be taken individually or combined. Glucosamine is an amino sugar that is produced by the body naturally and a precursor to a molecule called a glycosaminoglycan. This is used in the formation and repair of the cartilage that makes up the body's joints. Chondroitin is the most abundant glycosaminoglycan in cartilage, and is responsible for its resilience.

The ageing process can affect the body's ability to manufacture this vital compound, leading to the deterioration of weight-bearing joints. For this reason, glucosamine supplements have become increasingly popular as glucosamine is not readily available from primary food sources. Such supplements are available in a variety of forms: tablets, capsules, powders, skin patches or creams. Many are derived from animal tissue, particularly shellfish. Others, however, are produced by fermentation of grains such as corn or wheat.

Side-effects can occur, particularly within the digestive system. These include nausea, diarrhoea, constipation, indigestion and heartburn. Those with an allergy to shellfish should check the source of any supplement they are about to take.

Isoflavones

The chemical structure of isoflavones is very similar to that of oestrogen. Depending on the type of oestrogen receptor on the cells, isoflavones may reduce or activate the activity of oestrogen. Isoflavones can compete with oestrogen for the same receptor sites, thereby decreasing the health risks of excess oestrogen. They can also increase the oestrogen activity. If, during menopause, the body's natural level of oestrogen drops, isoflavones can compensate for this by binding to the same receptor, thereby easing menopause symptoms.

Isoflavones are present in relatively large amounts in virtually all soy products, with the exception of soy-protein concentrate. Soy contains many types of isoflavones, but the most beneficial are said to be genistein and daidzein. These are lower serum lipids, anti-oestrogenic, and may aid the prevention of breast and prostate cancers.

Isoflavones are also present in Red Clover. The beneficial effect of Red Clover isoflavones is very similar to that found in soy isoflavones. Isoflavones from Red Clover may reduce menopausal symptoms and help maintain the density of the bones in both menopausal and pre-menopausal women. Isoflavones may increase the incidence of epithelial hyperplasia and cause goitre and hyperthyroidism.

Case studies

① Ann is a successful teacher but has suffered from painful periods since puberty. Sometimes she has had to take time off work. Her doctor has ruled out any medical abnormality. She is also in pain from a wisdom tooth, which she is due to have removed. A friend suggests that she visit an alternative therapist to seek help.

- Discuss the treatments that her therapist might suggest to her. What, if anything, should she avoid? Why?

② Martin works as a lorry driver for a major haulage company. He has done so since leaving school, and mostly enjoys the work. An increase in the volume of traffic and greater pressure to meet delivery deadlines, however, are causing him to feel anxious and lose sleep. His doctor has suggested a course of Valium, but Martin is concerned about possible side-effects and the dangers of addiction. He has recently become interested in the use of CAMs.

- Discuss any possible alternatives to Valium that Martin might find useful.

Key learning points

Introduction

➢ CAMs are increasingly used in Western health care, both alongside conventional medicines and independent of them.

The range, scope and use of complementary therapies

➢ Trying to understand the true nature of CAMs takes time, patience and an open mind, as they are based on a philosophy of health very different from our own.

←

Popular therapies

➢ Osteopathy and Chiropractic medicine are manipulative therapies that concentrate on the musculo-skeletal system.
➢ Massage is a generic term for a variety of techniques which work therapeutically on the soft tissues of the body.
➢ Aromatherapy is the systematic use of essential oils, extracted from a wide variety of plants and highly concentrated, to improve physical and mental well-being.
➢ Homeopathy works on the principle of 'like cures like': a substance which may cause symptoms leading to illness is used to alleviate those symptoms.
➢ Although others are available, perhaps the most widely used flower remedies are those developed by Dr Edward Bach in the 1930s.

The modern context

➢ Cocaine, morphine, anticoagulants and quinine are among the many drugs in use today based on plants and herbs.
➢ In 2011 the MHRA imposed a requirement that any company manufacturing and marketing herbal remedies must register their products with them.
➢ Following assessments for safety and quality, a product is given a THR number comparable to the PLN given to any licensed medicine.

When might herbal remedies be of use?

➢ In contemporary society they are often used to treat depression, hormonal problems, stress and other common, often chronic, health problems.

Choice of herbs, contraindications and drug interactions

➢ Several constituents in Echinacea, working together, are thought to stimulate production and function of white blood cells, especially phagacytosis.
➢ Ginkgo is best known for improving mental alertness, circulation to the extremities and sexual function.
➢ Black Cohosh has been used to relieve nerve-related pain such as sciatica and neuralgia. It is thought to clear mucous and has been used to treat coughs.
➢ Cranberry may be used to treat urinary tract infections.
➢ Milk Thistle has been used in Europe as a liver tonic and to treat a whole range of liver and gall bladder conditions. Its chemical components are now being shown to have a protective effect on liver cells.
➢ The berries of the Saw Palmetto are enriched with fatty acids and phytosterols. Extracts from these act to tone and strengthen the male reproductive system.
➢ St John's Wort has the active ingredients hypericin and hyperforin which influence neurotransmitters in the brain. It may boost levels of the so-called 'feel-good' chemical serotonins, and is used for its antidepressant qualities.

→

←

> ➢ Valerian-based sedatives are widely available in European pharmacies.
> ➢ The active ingredient of Evening Primrose oil is GLA, an essential fatty acid. The oil is used to ease joint inflammation.

Multiple choice questions

1 Which of the following essential oils may be used neat in some circumstances?

a) Lavender
b) Black Pepper
c) Geranium
d) Tea Tree

2 Which of these should be avoided if you are about to undergo surgery?

a) Ginger
b) Black Cohosh
c) St John's Wort
d) Milk Thistle

3 Which of these therapies aims to treat 'like with like'?

a) Acupuncture
b) Osteopathy
c) Homeopathy
d) Acupressure

4 Which of the following is it illegal to sell in the UK?

a) Kava kava
b) Valerian
c) Hawthorn
d) Ginseng

5 Which of these may adversely affect those allergic to shellfish?

a) St John's Wort
b) Glucosamines
c) Isoflavones
d) Cranberry

→

6 When purchasing herbs to self-medicate it is most important to check

a) The picture on the packet
b) The expiry date
c) The price
d) The manufacturer

7 To work legally in the UK, which of the following must be registered?

a) An osteopath
b) An acupuncturist
c) A masseur
d) A dietician

8 Which of the following is used to treat liver disorders?

a) Ginger
b) Ginseng
c) Black Cohosh
d) Milk Thistle

9 Which of these would be of no benefit if undergoing the menopause?

a) Ginseng
b) Red Clover
c) Black Cohosh
d) Isoflavones

10 Which flower remedy would be used to treat anxiety?

a) Honeysuckle
b) Elm
c) Rock rose
d) Aspen

Recommended further reading

Adams, J. and Tovey, P. (2007) *Complementary and Alternative Medicine in Nursing and Midwifery: Towards a Critical Social Science.* London: Routledge.

Duke Center for Integrative Medicine (2006) *The Encyclopedia of New Medicine, Conventional and Alternative Medicine for all Ages.* London: Index Books.

Parkes, J. and Padmore, S. (2011) Symptom management: complementary and alternative medicine/integrated health, in M.A. Baldwin and J. Woodhouse (eds) *Key Concepts in Palliative Care.* London: Sage.

RCN (Royal College of Nursing) (2003) *Complementary Therapies in Nursing, Midwifery and Health Visiting Practice.* London: RCN.

Snyder, M. and Lindquist, R. (2010) *Complementary and Alternative Therapies in Nursing.* New York: Springer.

Useful links

Ayervedic Practitioners Association: www.apa.uk.com

Complementary and Natural Healthcare Council: www.cnhc.org.uk.

British Acupuncture Council: www.acupuncture.org.uk.

The Bach Centre: www.bachcentre.com.

The Complementary Therapists Association: www.ctha.com.

The General Osteopathic Council: www.osteopathy.org.uk.

The Medicines and Healthcare products Regulatory Agency (MHRA): www.mhra.gov.uk.

The National Institute of Medical Herbalists: www.nimh.org.uk.

The Society of Homeopaths: www.homeopathy-soh.org.

Answers

Chapter 1

Case study ①, Mrs Walker

You may have included aspects of the following:

- Statins are a class of drug that lowers the level of cholesterol in the blood.
- Statins block the enzyme in the liver that is responsible for making cholesterol.
- They help prevent significant build-up of atheroma.
- They help prevent the complications of atherosclerosis (angina, heart attacks, stroke, intermittent claudication and death).
- Statins are usually well absorbed, given orally and prescribed to be taken last thing before going to bed.
- The most serious (but fortunately rare) side-effects are liver failure and rhabdomyolysis.
- Since rhabdomyolysis may be fatal, unexplained joint or muscle pain that occurs while taking statins should be reported to the doctor for evaluation.

Case study ②, Geoff

You may have included aspects of the following:

- GTN belongs to a group of drugs called nitrates that contain the chemical nitric oxide.
- Nitric oxide is made naturally by the body and has the effect of making the veins and arteries relax and widen (dilate).
- More oxygen can be carried in the blood and the heart does not have to work so hard to keep up with both the demands of the tissues and the resistance caused by the atheroma in the vessels.

- Widening the veins also decreases the volume of blood that returns to the heart with each heartbeat (preload).
- GTN also widens the arteries within the heart itself, which increases the blood and oxygen supply to the heart muscle.
- The spray is applied under the tongue, as this area is highly vascular and avoids the first pass effect.
- Light-headedness or dizziness may be experienced especially when getting up from a sitting or lying position.
- Headaches are a possible side-effect as are fast or fluttering heartbeat, feeling sick and flushing.

Calculations

1. $30/60 \times 1 = 0.5$ tablets
2. Convert 0.25mg to mcg $= 250$
   $250/125 \times 1 = 2$ tablets
3. $125/50 \times 1ml = 2.5ml$
4. $6 \times 7 = 42$ tablets
5. $62.5/50 \times 1ml = 1.25ml$
6. $4/50 \times 100ml = 8ml/hr$
7. $25mcg \times 60 = 1500mcg$; convert to mg
   $1500/1000 = 1.5mg$
   $1.5/50 \times 50ml = 1.5ml/hr$
8. $400/200 \times 35ml = 70mg$
9. $1000/5 = 200ml$
10. Convert 0.1mg into mcg $0.1 \times 1000 = 100mcg$
    $100/50 \times 1ml = 2ml$

Multiple choice questions

1. b
2. d
3. a
4. a
5. d
6. c

7 b
8 d
9 c
10 d

Chapter 2

Case study ①, Mrs Johnson

You may have included aspects of the following:

- PPIs work by inhibiting gastric acid by blocking the H+/K+ ATP enzyme system (the proton pump) of the gastric parietal cell.
- PPIs have the potential to cause an increase in the prevalence of pneumonia and *Campylobacter enteritis* as well as doubling the risk of infection from *Clostridium difficile*. They have also been implicated in the increased rate of hip fractures, possibly due to altered calcium absorption. Rarer conditions such as nephritis and osteoporosis have also been documented.
- Aspects of Mrs Johnson's BMI need discussing related to her eating patterns. Smoking, alcohol and obesity are the most common risk factors in the overproduction of acidity leading to acid reflux. By reducing weight to within the recommended kilos for her height many symptoms can be reduced or eradicated. A healthy diet and lifestyle should be recommended.

Case study ②, Jack

You may have included aspects of the following:

- Crohn's disease is considered to be an autoimmune disease whereby the body's immune system attacks the GI tract, which ultimately causes inflammation. There has been evidence to suggest a genetic link to the disease, highlighting the risks to individuals and siblings and that males and females are equally affected.
- Prednisolone is a synthetic compound which mimics the actions of corticosteroids and has an anti-inflammatory and immunosuppressive quality. It is used until remission occurs at

which point it is withdrawn in reducing doses over a period of days.
- Mesalazine is given to relieve symptoms during an acute attack of mainly ulcerative colitis, and is also used in the treatment of Crohn's disease.
- Jack should be aware that the incidence of the disease is twofold in people who smoke.

Calculations

1   $1^1/_2$ tablets $= 1 \times 150$mg tablet, $^1/_2$ tablet $=$ 75mg, 150mg $+$ 75mg $=$ 225mg
2   4 tablets
    4×5mg $= 20$mg
3   8 tablets
    15mg $\times 2 = 30$mg
    $2 \times 4 = 8$ tablets
4   40ml
    10ml $\times 4 = 40$ml
5   2400mg
    400mg $\times 6 = 2400$mg
6   6 hourly
7   5 injections
    100mg $\div$ 20mg/ml $= 5$ injections
8   100mg/hr
    2.4g divided into 24 $= 100$mg/hr
9   20ml
    1g $= 5$ml
    $5 \times 4 = 20$ml
10 3 capsules
    0.6ml $\div$ 0.2ml $= 3$

Multiple choice questions

1   d
2   c
3   b
4   c
5   d
6   a
7   b
8   b
9   d
10 b

Chapter 3

Case study ①, the nurse

You may have included aspects of the following:

- Cyclophosphamide is an example of an alkylating agent which works directly on the DNA and prevents the cell division process.
- Alkylating drugs are effective during all phases of the cell cycle.
- Doxorubicin, which is a commonly used anthracycline chemotherapy agent, is isolated from a mutated strain of *Streptomyces*. These compounds are cell-cycle non-specific (i.e. they are effective during all phases of the cell cycle).
- Anthracyclines work by forming free radicals. These break DNA strands thereby inhibiting DNA production and function.
- Fluorouracil is a pyrimidine antagonist which acts to block the synthesis of pyrimidine-containing nucleotides (cytosine and thymine in DNA; cytosine and uracil in RNA).

Case study ②, Zachary

You may have included aspects of the following:

- Goserelin stops the production of leuteinizing hormone by the pituitary gland. This reduces the production of testosterone in men.
- The cancer may often shrink in size.
- Goserelin is given as an injection every 4 weeks, or as a longer-acting preparation every 12 weeks.
- The injection is often referred to as an 'implant' and the drug is mixed with oil so that the injections last over a period of time.
- Side-effects include tumour flare and Zachary may experience an increase in bone pain or have problems passing urine. Other problems may occasionally occur due to a temporary increase in the size of the tumour. If Zachary experiences any of these problems he should tell his doctor immediately.
- Loss of sex drive (libido) and erection difficulties (impotence) can occur. These effects often

return to normal after stopping the drug. There may also be an increased risk of developing heart disease or diabetes; however, the benefits far outweigh the risks involved in taking this medication.

Calculations

1	21 drops/min
2	75 min
3	17 drops/min
4	3mg
5	300mcg
6	46mg
7	0.7mg
8	330mcg
9	3.75ml
10	2hr 30min

Multiple choice questions

1	a
2	c
3	d
4	b
5	c
6	a
7	d
8	c
9	d
10	c

Chapter 4

Case study ①, the senior student

You may have included aspects of the following:

- Cyclizine is an antihistamine.
- It affects the CTZ and blocks histamine from triggering the vomiting reflex.
- Cyclizine may be given orally as 50mg tablets three times daily.

- If the patient is nauseous and vomiting it may be given as an IM or IV injection of 50mg up to three times daily.
- In children of 6–12 years the dose is halved to 25mg three times daily.
- Side-effects include drowsiness and sedation in many patients, therefore they should be warned about using machinery or driving while taking this medicine.
- Cardiovascular side-effects can include hypotension, tachycardia and palpitations.
- The drug is not given to patients with closed angle glaucoma or prostatic enlargement (hypertrophy).

Case study ②, Ménière's disease sufferer

You may have included aspects of the following:

- Betahistine is a medicine that closely resembles the natural substance histamine.
- It is often promoted as the specific treatment for the disease, especially in the UK.
- The medicine comes as a tablet in either an 8 or 16mg dose. Initially the patient would receive a dose of 16mg three times daily.
- As symptoms lessen the patient should be stabilized on a dose of 24–48mg daily.
- Betahistine works by reducing the pressure of the fluid that fills the labyrinth in the inner ear.

Calculations

1   42 drops/min
2   0.8ml
3   Half a tablet
4   1ml
5   7.5ml
6   1.25ml
7   2ml
8   Half a tablet
9   45ml in 24hr
10 16mg

Multiple choice questions

1   d
2   b
3   c·
4   a
5   a
6   c
7   d
8   b
9   b
10 d

Chapter 5

Case study ①, Hamza

You may have included aspects of the following:

- Hamza had local anaesthetic 'patches' on each hand so that he wouldn't feel the cannula being inserted. Both hands are treated in case cannulation is difficult in one, or both need cannulating.
- Propofol for induction. Sevoflurane in O_2 and air for maintenance. Paracetamol, diclofenac and morphine for analgesia.
- Dexamethasone and ondansetron.

Case study ②, Abbi

You may have included aspects of the following:

- Abbi was given fentanyl prior to induction to provide analgesia.
- Abbi was having major surgery therefore an endotracheal tube was required to facilitate artificial ventilation.
- Rocuronium is a competitive neuromuscular (non-depolarizing) agent.
- Rocuronium may still be working at the end of the surgery so Abbi would wake up still paralysed unless the effects of the NMB were reversed. Glycopyrronium bromide is given with neostigmine to prevent bradycardia, excessive salivation and other muscarinic effects of neostigmine.

Multiple choice questions

1   b
2   c
3   c
4   a, d
5   b, d
6   c
7   b
8   d
9   c
10 b

Chapter 6

Case study ①, explaining natural immunity

You may have included aspects of the following:

- Following the birth of a baby the mother produces colostrum as part of the breast milk, which is rich in antibodies that reflect the mother's own immunity.
- Colostrum is low in fat, high in carbohydrates, protein and, in particular, secretory immunoglobulin G (IgG).
- After birth another antibody (IgA) protects the baby's mucous membranes in the throat, lung and intestines.
- Colostrum seals the holes in the GI tract by coating it with a barrier which prevents foreign substances from penetrating.
- Colostrum acts as a laxative which helps to clean out meconium, which in turn decreases the likelihood of jaundice in the baby.
- Breastfeeding offers protection to the baby for the duration of the feeding programme. The mother continues to pass antibodies in breast milk after the colostrum is depleted (about 10–14 days) and the mature milk is present.

Case study ②, explaining active immunity

You may have included aspects of the following:

- Vaccines are designed to trigger the immune system to produce its own antibodies against disease.
- Vaccination entails the introduction of a foreign molecule into the body, which causes the body to generate immunity against it.
- The direct action of antibodies makes the body think it has been infected with the disease itself.
- Immunity comes from lymphocytes (made in the bone marrow) which are subdivided into B-cell and T-cell types.
- The immune system is very efficient in recognizing and destroying the microbe if the body is re-exposed to it.
- The immune system produces memory cells which trigger the immune response very quickly should the person be exposed to the disease again.

Multiple choice questions

1   d
2   a
3   c
4   d
5   b
6   c
7   a
8   b
9   c
10 b

Chapter 7

Case study ①, Simon

You may have included aspects of the following:

- An open fracture of the femur carries the risk of severe bleeding. A patient may lose up to a litre of blood or more from the broken femur bone. This equates to losing 20 per cent of total blood circulating volume which is an emergency situation. Simon's blood pressure is dropping as a result. Gelofusine is a plasma enhancer and has large molecules that do not readily cross capillary membranes so that they are retained in the blood vessels, which helps to maintain blood pressure. Normal saline 0.9 per cent (crystalloid) has much smaller molecules and is rapidly absorbed into the interstitial spaces; this only gives between 30–60 minutes of blood volume replacement. Less gelofusine will be needed to maintain Simon's blood pressure. In addition, administering gelofusine is less likely to cause fluid overload. The action of gelofusine can last for a number of days whereas the action of a crystalloid only lasts for a number of minutes or hours. If cross-matching for blood is required gelofusine supports the body's blood pressure while the correct cross-match is achieved.

● Simon's vital signs and symptoms are all signs that blood is being diverted from the peripheries (arms, legs and skin) to maintain core pressure (heart, lungs and brain). His confusion and disorientation are likely to be due to decreased cerebral perfusion and hypoxia. Hypotension will result from the decreased circulatory volume of blood. An increased heart rate is the result of the heart having to beat faster to circulate the now compromised reduced blood volume due to the open fracture. Increased respirations are also in response to the reduced amount of blood in the circulating volume. As blood volume is lost so are the oxygen-carrying red blood cells that maintain the oxygenation of all cells within homeostasis. Simon's shaking could be a sign of hypothermia due to the evaporation of sweat. He is also at risk of developing fluid-induced hypothermia where his core temperature falls below 37 degrees due to the cold fluid being administered.

Case study ②, patient with painful hand

You may have included aspects of the following:

● The tip of the cannula may have withdrawn or become dislodged from the vein, or protruded through the vein into the surrounding tissue allowing fluid/blood to seep in. Thus the cannula has 'tissued' resulting in infiltration.

As the patient is elderly, her veins are likely to be fragile and quite thready. The blanching (whiteness) around the cannula site and cold skin are signs of transient ischaemia (deficient blood supply to any part of the body). The patient's hand is cold due to IV fluid seeping into the subcutaneous tissue around the cannula site.

● You should stop the IV infusion immediately, remove the cannula and make arrangements for it to be re-sited. To provide symptomatic relief, apply either a cold or a hot compress to ease discomfort. Reassure the patient about what has happened and explain that a new cannula will need to be sited. Answer any questions she has regarding this. Document the incident in her care plan and continue to monitor the original cannula site for signs of infection.

Calculations

1   455ml
2   300ml
3   60ml
4   40 drops per min
5   10 drops per min
6   150 drops per min
7   63 drops per min
8   300 min
9   13 drops per min
10   100 min

Multiple choice questions

1   b
2   b
3   d
4   c
5   d
6   d
7   a
8   c
9   c
10   a

Chapter 8

Case study ①, Philip

You may have included aspects of the following:

- Philip needs to recommence his emollient therapy. Emollients are moisturizers that soothe by preventing water loss from skin. They will reduce the dryness of his skin and ease itching. This will help to prevent the flare-ups of eczema.
- Emollients are most effective at alleviating eczema when they are used frequently, even when the patient doesn't have eczema symptoms. Therefore you will need to consider educating Philip so that he understands the need to use his creams as prescribed.
- Steroid cream such as hydrocortisone, which reduces inflammation and helps to relieve itching, may be considered. There are different strength steroid creams available. Mild steroid creams can be purchased over the counter. Philip's parents should be advised to ask their pharmacist for advice. Stronger steroid creams, such as betamethasone are available on prescription. However, using them too often, or on delicate skin (such as the face), can thin the skin. This could make Philip's skin bruise more easily. His parents should be advised to always follow their GP's guidance concerning steroid creams. If emollients or steroid creams don't help Philip's eczema, there is a range of other medicines his GP may prescribe such as topical immunosuppressants. Oral steroids, such as prednisolone, are available as tablets to treat severe eczema but should only be used as a last resort.

Case study ②, Bilal

You may have included aspects of the following:

- Scabies.
- You may recommend permethrin 5 per cent to be painted over the whole body, paying particular attention to the webs of the fingers and toes and under the nails. This should be washed off after 8–12 hours and then repeated after seven days.
- Advise that itching may continue for some time after treatment.

Calculations

1   0.5ml in 100ml of solution
2   1mg
3   0.125g
4   2 per cent
5   1 in 200
6   0.5mg/ml
7   56 tablets
8   30 finger tip units
9   1.005kg
10   5ml of 10 per cent solution with 45ml diluent

Multiple choice questions

1   d
2   c
3   a
4   a
5   a
6   b
7   b
8   a
9   d
10   c

Chapter 9

Case study ①, NRT therapies

You may have included aspects of the following:

- Nicotine gum. Two strengths are available, 2mg and 4mg. The 4mg strength should be used if the person smokes 18 or more cigarettes a day. After two to three months the individual should be using the gum less and less.
- Nicotine patches. Some patches last 16 hours and are only worn when awake; others last 24 hours and are worn the whole time. They

are discreet and easy to apply but only a steady amount of nicotine is delivered.

- Nicotine inhalers resemble a cigarette into which a cartridge is inserted and inhaled in an action similar to smoking. They are especially suitable for patients who miss the hand-to-mouth movements of smoking.
- Tablets and lozenges are designed to be dissolved under the tongue whereby nicotine is absorbed through the mouth into the bloodstream. Very easy to use.
- Nasal spray. The nicotine in the spray is rapidly absorbed into the bloodstream from the nose and this form of NRT most closely mimics the rapid increase in nicotine level that a person gets from smoking a cigarette. Side-effects include nose and throat irritation, coughing and watering eyes.

Case study ②, use of disulfiram

You may have included aspects of the following:

- Disulfiram (Antabuse) is helpful in maintaining abstinence and leads to an accumulation of the intermediary alcoholic metabolic product, acetaldehyde, when alcohol is consumed. The result is flushing, dyspnoea, palpitations, nausea and hypotension. Patients should be advised of these unpleasant effects before the medicine is commenced. It is important to be vigilant for any severe reaction. The patient should not normally take this medication for longer than a six-month period.

Calculations

1   4 tablets
2   6 tablets
3   20ml
4   1920mcg
5   15 pieces
6   0.5mg
7   2.8mg
8   12 tablets
9   40mg
10 100mg on two days and 150mg on one day

Multiple choice questions

1   a
2   c
3   d
4   a
5   c
6   d
7   b
8   b
9   d
10 a

Chapter 10

Case study ①, Ann

You may have included aspects of the following:

- Following a discussion of her medical history and symptoms Ann's therapist might suggest a course of either Ginkgo Biloba or Black Cohosh. Both would be effective in treating premenstrual symptoms and painful periods. Ginkgo, however, promotes bleeding, and should be avoided by those about to undergo surgery or dental treatment. Black Cohosh does not promote bleeding, but should be avoided by those who are pregnant. As Ann is not pregnant, a course of Black Cohosh would seem appropriate.

Case study ②, Martin

You may have included aspects of the following:

- Martin could visit a local pharmacy and discuss what alternatives are available. St John's Wort can be purchased over the counter and could prove beneficial. Alternatively, he could visit a therapist to discuss other options, possibly reflexology or aromatherapy. An appropriate Bach remedy may prove helpful. Aspen is thought to counter feelings of anxiety.

Multiple choice questions

1   a, d
2   a
3   c
4   a

5   b
6   b
7   a
8   d
9   b
10 d

Index

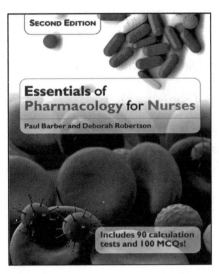

ESSENTIALS OF PHARMACOLOGY FOR NURSES 2/E

Paul Barber and Deborah Robertson

9780335245659 (Paperback)
May 2012

eBook also available

This popular book introduces pharmacology and calculations in a friendly, informative way and is now updated throughout with new topics and new coverage of more drugs and drug issues. The book focuses on the pharmacology knowledge needed at pre-registration level and does not assume previous knowledge of pharmacology, or a level of confidence with maths and drugs calculations.

Key features:

- Calculation sections containing 90 calculations to help perfect calculation skills
- 100 multiple choice questions to help the reader assess learning
- Patient scenarios from a range of different clinical settings, demonstrating pharmacology in clinical settings

www.openup.co.uk

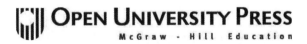

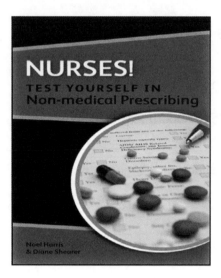

NURSES! TEST YOURSELF IN NON-MEDICAL PRESCRIBING

Noel Harris and Diane Shearer

9780335244997 (Paperback)
August 2012

eBook also available

Part of the 'Nurses! Test yourself in..' series, this book covers the main topics from non-medical prescribing courses and modules that appear in the exam. This includes pharmacology and calculations as well as the legal, procedural and practical aspects of the prescribing role that are assessed on the course such as: drug safety, consultation skills, adverse drug reactions, concordance, using the BNF and special care groups such as children, pregnant women and mental health clients.

Key features:

- A range of question types, including True or False and Multiple Choice
- Questions based around mini-case scenarios for prescribing
- Provides a list of clearly explained answers to questions, so the book can be used as a 'teach and test' resource

www.openup.co.uk

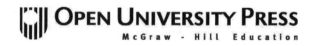

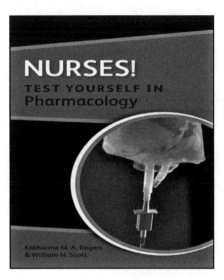

NURSES! TEST YOURSELF IN PHARMACOLOGY

Katherine Rogers and William Scott

9780335244911 (Paperback)
August 2012

eBook also available

Part of the '*Nurses! Test yourself in..*' series, this book is designed as a revision and study aid for student nurses undertaking their pharmacology module/s and related exam assessment. Containing both self-assessment questions and quizzes, this book will test students learning and help them tackle their knowledge gaps by explaining the answers to all the featured questions.

Key features:

- Organised into body systems chapters
- Includes a range of question types
- Provides a list of clearly explained answers to questions

www.openup.co.uk

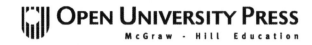

OPEN UNIVERSITY PRESS
McGraw - Hill Education

The **McGraw·Hill** Companies

What's new from Open University Press?

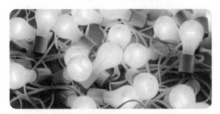
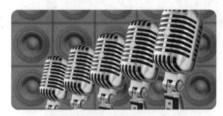

Education... Media, Film & Cultural Studies

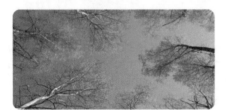
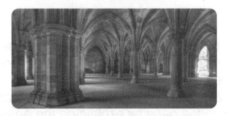

Health, Nursing & Social Welfare... Higher Education

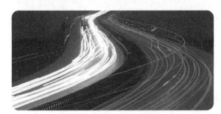
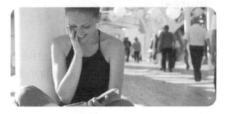

Psychology, Counselling & Psychotherapy... Study Skills

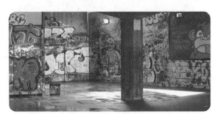

Keep up with what's buzzing
at Open University Press
by signing up to receive
regular title information at
www.openup.co.uk/elert

Sociology

OPEN UNIVERSITY PRESS

McGraw - Hill Education